T0263339

Endoscopic Submucosal Dissection

Editor

NORIO FUKAMI

GASTROINTESTINAL ENDOSCOPY CLINICS OF NORTH AMERICA

www.giendo.theclinics.com

Consulting Editor
CHARLES J. LIGHTDALE

April 2014 • Volume 24 • Number 2

ELSEVIER

1600 John F. Kennedy Boulevard • Suite 1800 • Philadelphia, Pennsylvania, 19103-2899

http://www.theclinics.com

**GASTROINTESTINAL ENDOSCOPY CLINICS OF NORTH AMERICA Volume 24, Number 2
April 2014 ISSN 1052-5157, ISBN-13: 978-0-323-29484-3**

Editor: Kerry Holland
Developmental Editor: Donald Mumford

Gastrointestinal Endoscopy Clinics of North America (ISSN 1052-5157) is published quarterly by Elsevier Inc., 360 Park Avenue South, New York, NY 10010-1710. Months of issue are January, April, July, and October. Business and Editorial Offices: 1600 John F. Kennedy Blvd., Suite 1800, Philadelphia, PA, 19103-2899. Periodicals postage paid at New York, NY and additional mailing offices. Subscription prices are $335.00 per year for US individuals, $486.00 per year for US institutions, $175.00 per year for US students and residents, $370.00 per year for Canadian individuals, $576.00 per year for Canadian institutions, $465.00 per year for international individuals, $576.00 per year for international institutions, and $245.00 per year for Canadian and foreign students/residents. To receive student/resident rate, orders must be accompanied by name of affiliated institution, date of term, and the *signature* of program/residency coordinator on institution letterhead. Orders will be billed at individual rate until proof of status is received. Foreign air speed delivery is included in all *Clinics* subscription prices. All prices are subject to change without notice. **POSTMASTER:** Send address change to *Gastrointestinal Endoscopy Clinics of North America*, Elsevier Health Sciences Division, Subscription Customer Service, 3251 Riverport Lane, Maryland Heights, MO 63043. **Customer Service: 1-800-654-2452 (US). From outside the United States, call 1-314-447-8871. Fax: 1-314-447-8029. E-mail: JournalsCustomerService-usa@elsevier.com (for print support) or JournalsOnlineSupport-usa@elsevier.com (for online support).**

Reprints. For copies of 100 or more, of articles in this publication, please contact the Commercial Reprints Department, Elsevier Inc., 360 Park Avenue South, New York, NY 10010-1710. Tel. 212-633-3874; Fax: 212-633-3820; E-mail: reprints@elsevier.com.

Gastrointestinal Endoscopy Clinics of North America is covered in *Excerpta Medica, MEDLINE/PubMed (Index Medicus), and MEDLINE/MEDLARS.*

Contributors

CONSULTING EDITOR

CHARLES J. LIGHTDALE, MD
Professor of Medicine, Department of Medicine, Columbia University Medical Center, New York, New York

EDITOR

NORIO FUKAMI, MD, AGAF, FACG, FASGE
Associate Professor of Medicine, Division of Gastroenterology and Hepatology, Director of Endoscopic Ultrasound, Innovative Technology, and Endoscopic Oncology, Medical Co-Director, Digestive Health Center, University of Colorado, Anschutz Medical Campus, Aurora, Colorado

AUTHORS

TAKESHI AZUMA, MD, PhD
Professor, Frontier Medical Science in Gastroenterology, Kobe University School of Medicine, Kobe, Hyogo, Japan

JOO YOUNG CHO, MD, PhD
Digestive Disease Center, Soonchunhyang University Hospital, Seoul, Korea

JUN-HYUNG CHO, MD
Digestive Disease Center, Soonchunhyang University Hospital, Seoul, Korea

PETER DRAGANOV, MD, PhD, FASGE
Professor, Division of Gastroenterology, Hepatology and Nutrition, University of Florida, Gainesville, Florida

NORIO FUKAMI, MD, AGAF, FACG, FASGE
Associate Professor of Medicine, Division of Gastroenterology and Hepatology, Director of Endoscopic Ultrasound, Innovative Technology, and Endoscopic Oncology, Medical Co-Director, Digestive Health Center, University of Colorado, Anschutz Medical Campus, Aurora, Colorado

CHRISTOPHER J. GOSTOUT, MD
Developmental Endoscopy Unit, Division of Gastroenterology and Hepatology, Mayo Clinic College of Medicine, Rochester, Minnesota

OSAMU GOTO, MD, PhD
Assistant Professor, Division of Research and Development for Minimally Invasive Treatment, Cancer Center, School of Medicine, Keio University, Shinjuku-ku, Tokyo, Japan

TAKUJI GOTODA, MD, PhD, FASGE, FRCP
Associate Professor, Department of Gastroenterology and Hepatology, Tokyo Medical University, Shinjuku-ku, Tokyo, Japan

KHEK-YU HO, MD, PhD
Professor, Department of Medicine, Yong Loo Lin School of Medicine, National University of Singapore, Singapore

JOICHIRO HORII, MD, PhD
Assistant Professor, Division of Research and Development for Minimally Invasive Treatment, Cancer Center, School of Medicine, Keio University, Shinjuku-ku, Tokyo, Japan

HARUHIRO INOUE, MD, PhD, FASGE
Professor and Director, Digestive Diseases Center, Showa University Koto-Toyosu Hospital, Tokyo, Japan

PANKAJ JAIN, MD
Department of Gastroenterology, Sterling Hospital, Vadodara, India

TONYA KALTENBACH, MD, MS, FASGE
Assistant Professor, Department of Gastroenterology and Hepatology, Veterans Affairs Palo Alto, Stanford University, Palo Alto, California

MI-YOUNG KIM, MD, PhD
Digestive Disease Center, Soonchunhyang University Hospital, Seoul, Korea

SHIN-EI KUDO, MD, PhD
Digestive Diseases Center, Showa University Koto-Toyosu Hospital, Tokyo, Japan

MARIKO MAN-I, MD, PhD
Doctor, Frontier Medical Science in Gastroenterology, Kobe University School of Medicine, Kobe, Hyogo, Japan

TAKAHISA MATSUDA, MD, PhD
Endoscopy Division, National Cancer Center Hospital, Chuo-ku, Tokyo, Japan

YOSHIMASA MIURA, MD
Senior Staff Specialist, Gastroenterology Center, Jichi Medical University, Shimotsuke, Tochigi, Japan

YOSHINORI MORITA, MD, PhD
Associate Professor, Department of Gastroenterology, Kobe University School of Medicine, Chuo-ku, Kobe, Hyogo, Japan

TAKESHI NAKAJIMA, MD, PhD
Endoscopy Division, National Cancer Center Hospital, Chuo-ku, Tokyo, Japan

HORST NEUHAUS, MD
Professor of Medicine, Head, Department of Internal Medicine, Evangelisches Krankenhaus Düsseldorf, Teaching Hospital of the University of Düsseldorf, Düsseldorf, Germany

TAKESHI OHKI, MD, PhD
Assistant Professor, Department of Surgery, Institute of Gastroenterology, Tokyo Women's Medical University; Institute of Advanced Biomedical Engineering and Science, Tokyo Women's Medical University (TWIns), Shinjuku-ku, Tokyo, Japan

TERUO OKANO, PhD
Professor, Institute of Advanced Biomedical Engineering and Science, Tokyo Women's Medical University (TWIns), Shinjuku-ku, Tokyo, Japan

MANABU ONIMARU, MD, PhD
Digestive Diseases Center, Showa University Koto-Toyosu Hospital, Tokyo, Japan

TSUNEO OYAMA, MD, PhD
Director, Department of Gastroenterology, Saku Central Hospital, Nagano, Japan

CHANG BEOM RYU, MD, PhD
Professor of Medicine, Gastroenterology Division, Soonchunhyang University College of Medicine, Digestive Disease Center and Research Institute, Sonnchunhyang University Bucheon Hospital, Bucheon, Gyeonggi-do, South Korea

YUTAKA SAITO, MD, PhD
Endoscopy Division, National Cancer Center Hospital, Chuo-ku, Tokyo, Japan

TAKU SAKAMOTO, MD
Endoscopy Division, National Cancer Center Hospital, Chuo-ku, Tokyo, Japan

ESPERANZA GRACE SANTI, MD, PhD
Section of Gastroenterology, Department of Internal Medicine, De La Salle University Medical Center, Manila, Philippines

ROY SOETIKNO, MD, MS, FASGE
Professor, Department of Gastroenterology and Hepatology, Veterans Affairs Palo Alto, Stanford University, Palo Alto, California

KAZUKI SUMIYAMA, MD, PhD
Department of Endoscopy, The Jikei University School of Medicine, Minato-ku, Tokyo, Japan

HISAO TAJIRI, MD, PhD
Department of Endoscopy; Division of Gastroenterology and Hepatology, Department of Internal Medicine, The Jikei University School of Medicine, Minato-ku, Tokyo, Japan

TAKASHI TOYONAGA, MD
Associate Professor, Department of Endoscopy, Kobe University Hospital, Kobe; Frontier Medical Science in Gastroenterology, Kobe University School of Medicine, Kobe, Hyogo, Japan

TOSHIO URAOKA, MD, PhD
Associate Professor, Division of Research and Development for Minimally Invasive Treatment, Cancer Center, School of Medicine, Keio University, Shinjuku-ku, Tokyo, Japan

NAOHISA YAHAGI, MD, PhD
Professor and Director, Division of Research and Development for Minimally Invasive Treatment, Cancer Center, School of Medicine, Keio University, Shinjuku-ku, Tokyo, Japan

HIRONORI YAMAMOTO, MD, PhD
Professor, Director of Gastroenterology Center, Jichi Medical University, Shimotsuke, Tochigi, Japan

MASAKAZU YAMAMOTO, MD, PhD
Professor, Department of Surgery, Institute of Gastroenterology, Tokyo Women's Medical University, Shinjuku-ku, Tokyo, Japan

MASAYUKI YAMATO, PhD
Professor, Institute of Advanced Biomedical Engineering and Science, Tokyo Women's Medical University (TWIns), Shinjuku-ku, Tokyo, Japan

Contents

Endoscopic resection is now considered a curative procedure for early gastric cancer. In Japan, it has increasingly replaced surgical resection for this indication, although in the West it has not been universally accepted as a first-line treatment. Recently, endoscopic submucosal dissection has been increasingly applied to colorectal disease, although it has not become a standard therapeutic procedure for early colorectal carcinoma because of its technical difficulty, the relatively long procedure time required, and the risk of complications, such as perforation and bleeding.

Endoscopic submucosal dissection (ESD) is useful for submucosal tumors (SMTs) within the superficial submucosal layer, but perforation frequently occurs during ESD for SMTs located at the deeper layer. Endoscopic resection for small esophageal SMTs is acceptable, although candidates for endoscopic removal are rare. Laparoscopic assistance will be effective for minimally invasive endoscopic local resection for certain types of gastric SMT. Endoscopic mucosal resection with a ligation device would be better than ESD for rectal carcinoid in terms of simplicity and effectiveness.

 A case presentation of electrocautery for ESD accompanies this article

An electrical surgical unit (ESU) performs incisions and coagulation through applying Joule heat, generated by a high-frequency current onto tissue without neuromuscular stimulation. Output by the ESU includes incision output and coagulation output. Incision output is needed to generate a steam explosion (spark) by quickly increasing the intracellular fluid temperature through continuous application of Joule heat generated by the high-frequency current (unmodulated pulse: continuous wave). To perform safe and successful endoscopic submucosal dissection, one must fully understand the principles and features of an ESU to use settings

complications, delayed bleeding, and perforation. A small-caliber-tip transparent hood is useful. Mechanical stretching of the submucosal tissue allows safe dissection and effective prevention of bleeding with minimum muscle injury under direct visualization of the submucosal tissue and blood vessels. A short double-balloon endoscope is useful to stabilize control of the endoscope tip in distal duodenal ESD. Selection of ESD in the duodenum should be made cautiously considering both benefits and risks of the procedure.

Colorectal ESD: Current Indications and Latest Technical Advances

Yutaka Saito, Taku Sakamoto, Takeshi Nakajima, and Takahisa Matsuda

The number of medical facilities that perform colorectal endoscopic submucosal dissection (ESD) has been growing, and its effectiveness has been increasingly reported in recent years. Indications approved by the Japanese government's medical insurance system are early colorectal cancers with a maximum tumor size of 2–5 cm. ESD was an effective procedure for treating noninvasive colorectal tumors difficult to resect en bloc by conventional EMR, resulting in a higher en bloc resection rate that is less invasive than surgery. Based on the excellent clinical results of colorectal ESDs, the Japanese health care insurance system has approved colorectal ESD for coverage.

Submucosal Endoscopy: From ESD to POEM and Beyond

Haruhiro Inoue, Esperanza Grace Santi, Manabu Onimaru, and Shin-ei Kudo

Peroral endoscopic myotomy (POEM) is an evolving minimally invasive endoscopic surgical procedure, with no skin incision, intended for long-term recovery from symptoms of esophageal achalasia. POEM was developed based on both the already established surgical principles of esophageal myotomy and the advanced techniques of endoscopic submucosal dissection. This article relates how POEM was developed, and its use in practice is reported and discussed. As an extension of the POEM technique, submucosal endoscopic tumor resection is introduced.

Investigating Deeper: Muscularis Propria to Natural Orifice Transluminal Endoscopic Surgery

Kazuki Sumiyama, Christopher J. Gostout, and Hisao Tajiri

Submucosal endoscopy with a mucosal flap (SEMF) safety valve technique is a global concept in which the submucosa is a free working space for endoscopic interventions. A purposefully created intramural space provides an endoscopic access route to the deeper layers and into the extraluminal cavities. The mucosa overlying the intramural space is protective, reducing contamination during natural orifice transluminal endoscopic surgery (NOTES) procedures and providing a sealant flap to repair the entry point and the submucosal space. In addition to NOTES, SEMF enables endoscopic achalasia myotomy, histologic analysis of the muscularis propria, and submucosal tumor removal.

candidate lesions in the gastrointestinal tract, and adequate training programs. Yet American physicians are becoming increasingly aware of the
benefits of ESD. Simplification of technique, modification of tools and materials, and improved availability of training opportunities are essential in
order to accelerate the adoption of ESD in the United States.

GASTROINTESTINAL ENDOSCOPY CLINICS OF NORTH AMERICA

ISSUE OF RELATED INTEREST

Gastroenterology Clinics of North America, June 2013 (Vol. 43, No. 2)
Gastric Cancer
Steven Moss, MD, *Guest Editor*

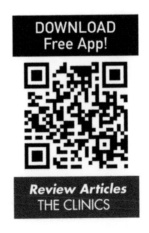

**DOWNLOAD
Free App!**

Review Articles
THE CLINICS

NOW AVAILABLE FOR YOUR iPhone and iPad

Foreword

Endoscopic Submucosal Dissection: On the Rise from East to West

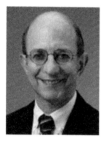

Charles J. Lightdale, MD
Consulting Editor

In the history of gastrointestinal endoscopy, every once in a while a new therapeutic method comes to the fore that seems difficult and risky, yet so elegant and dramatic in its benefits and possibilities that it fires the desire of interventional endoscopists worldwide to perform it. One such technique is endoscopic submucosal dissection (ESD), the subject of this issue of the *Gastrointestinal Endoscopy Clinics of North America*. ESD has been developed in Japan and is now rapidly spreading around the globe. The initial indication was to resect early gastric cancers en bloc to decrease recurrence. From there, ESD has been utilized from the esophagus to the colon for en-bloc resection of early cancers. The procedure has also opened up the submucosal space for other therapeutic measures, including resection of subepithelial tumors, and most notably for per-oral endoscopic myotomy for achalasia. Other variations useful for natural orifice transluminal endoscopic surgery are being perfected.

We can only be grateful to the Japanese innovators who have so generously given their time and effort to train a first wave of international practitioners of ESD. During the Peter D. Stevens Course on Innovations in Digestive Care at the New York-Presbyterian Hospital in 2012, I stood next to a young master endoscopist, Norio Fukami, from the University of Colorado, as he performed an ESD procedure in a live demonstration with a calm ease that took my breath away. That same day I asked if he would be willing to be guest editor for an issue of the *Gastrointestinal Endoscopy Clinics of North America* on ESD, and he immediately accepted. He has gathered an extraordinary group of pioneering experts from Japan as well as others from the United States

Gastrointest Endoscopy Clin N Am 24 (2014) xiii–xiv
http://dx.doi.org/10.1016/j.giec.2014.02.001
1052-5157/14/$ – see front matter © 2014 Published by Elsevier Inc.

giendo.theclinics.com

and Europe to produce a landmark volume (with videos) on ESD, which should be pored over and treasured as the premier and comprehensive guide to this important new method in therapeutic gastrointestinal endoscopy.

Charles J. Lightdale, MD
Department of Medicine
Columbia University Medical Center
161 Fort Washington Avenue, Room 812
New York, NY 10032, USA

E-mail address:
CJL18@columbia.edu

Preface

Endoscopic Submucosal Dissection

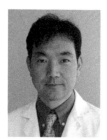

Norio Fukami, MD, AGAF, FACG, FASGE
Editor

The innovative procedure, later named endoscopic submucosal dissection (ESD), was invented in Japan in the late 1990s to address the existing limitations of and to expand endoscopic treatment of early gastric cancer. Multiple Japanese physicians modified the available equipment and techniques to perfect the procedure and improve outcomes over the past decade, and now ESD is performed in nearly all segments of the gastrointestinal tract and is practiced in many countries. Moreover, the indications of ESD are ever expanding due to further refinement of the technique and as we learn more about the evidence related to excellent outcomes of patients treated by this procedure. ESD has benefited many patients who were diagnosed with an early stage of gastrointestinal cancer, and this has prompted a significant worldwide demand to learn more about its indications, technical aspects, and outcomes to adopt ESD in major academic medical centers and possibly even individual physicians' practices for the benefit of patients.

In this issue of *Gastrointestinal Endoscopy Clinics of North America*, we invited pioneers and experts in this field to share recent advancements and expansions of ESD and its technical aspects in different organ systems. In addition, this issue covers the associated techniques of per oral endoscopic myotomy (POEM) and natural orifice transluminal endoscopic surgery (NOTES) to further advance understanding of the latest breakthroughs in endoscopic therapy. Current trends surrounding ESD around the world—in Asia, Europe, and the United States—are addressed as well.

Some articles include videos for readers to watch ESD procedures in action, performed by experts, for easier understanding of ESD techniques. I have no doubt that this issue will inspire more physicians to explore the expanding possibilities of endoscopic therapy such as ESD and POEM and to advocate minimally invasive treatment for patients.

Gastrointest Endoscopy Clin N Am 24 (2014) xv–xvi
http://dx.doi.org/10.1016/j.giec.2014.01.001
1052-5157/14/$ – see front matter © 2014 Elsevier Inc. All rights reserved.

giendo.theclinics.com

I would like to thank all the authors for their excellent contributions that make this issue a comprehensive review and update for all physicians who are eager to learn ESD. Also, I would like to express my gratitude to Dr. Charles J. Lightdale, whose vision and inspiring leadership made this issue possible, and Kerry K. Holland, Senior Editor of Elsevier, for her effort and dedication to this issue. Last, I conclude with my gratitude to Alissa Bults, MS, whose assistance was vital to the success of this issue.

Norio Fukami, MD, AGAF, FACG, FASGE
Division of Gastroenterology and Hepatology, Therapeutic Endoscopy
University of Colorado
12631 East 17th Avenue, B158
Aurora, CO 80045, USA

E-mail address:
Norio.Fukami@UCDenver.edu

Expanding Indications for ESD
Mucosal Disease (Upper and Lower Gastrointestinal Tract)

Chang Beom Ryu, MD, PhD

KEYWORDS

- Endoscopic mucosal resection • Endoscopic submucosal dissection
- Early colorectal carcinoma • Early gastric cancer

KEY POINTS

- Experience with endoscopic resection of early gastric cancer has been recorded in various studies.
- Expansion of the criteria for endoscopic mucosal resection will reduce the need for gastrectomy in early gastric cancer.
- Although endoscopic submucosal dissection has been increasingly applied to colorectal disease, it has not become a standard therapeutic procedure for early colorectal carcinoma because of its technical difficulty; the relatively long procedure time required; and the risk of complications, such as perforation and bleeding.
- To help overcome the learning curve of colorectal endoscopic submucosal dissection, Western and Eastern endoscopic societies should communicate with each other.

UPPER GASTROINTESTINAL TRACT

Endoscopic resection is now considered a curative procedure for early gastric cancer. In Japan, it has increasingly replaced surgical resection for this indication, although in the West it has not been universally accepted as a first-line treatment. Endoscopic resection also has been used as a histologic staging technique for early gastric cancer by assessing the depth of tumor penetration, which is important in determining the best treatment.

Limited invasion of the tumor and absence of lymph node metastases are crucial for achieving a cure of gastric cancer with endoscopic therapy. The important endoscopic points to consider are as follows:

1. The extent of the surface involvement and the morphology. Endoscopic mucosal resection (EMR) is not recommended for lesions greater than 2 cm in size.

Gastroenterology Division, Soonchunhyang University College of Medicine, Digestive Disease Center and Research Institute, Sonnchunhyang University Bucheon Hospital, 1174 Jungdong, Wonmigu, Bucheon, Gyeonggi-do 420-767, South Korea
E-mail addresses: RyuChB@schbc.ac.kr; ryuchb@gmail.com

Gastrointest Endoscopy Clin N Am 24 (2014) 161–167
http://dx.doi.org/10.1016/j.giec.2013.12.002
1052-5157/14/$ – see front matter © 2014 Elsevier Inc. All rights reserved.

Endoscopic submucosal dissection (ESD) is recommend for lesions up to 3 cm if they are not ulcerated or scarred, or are less than 2 cm if they have ulcers or scars.

2. The depth of invasion should not be deeper than the mucosa or the most superficial submucosal layer, the upper third of the submucosa (sm1). The depth may be determined by endoscopic ultrasound examination before endoscopic resection, and corroborated with histopathologic examination of the resected specimen.

3. High-grade dysplasia is the earliest stage of malignancy. A high degree of cellular differentiation favors endoscopic treatment. Even though poorly differentiated lesions have a higher risk of distant spread, those less than 5 mm can be treated endoscopically.[1]

4. Multifocal early gastric cancer can be treated endoscopically provided the entire lesion is histologically consistent with intramucosal cancer.[2] The degree of difficulty in performing endoscopic resection depends in part on the location of the tumor in the stomach; lesions in the posterior wall and lesser curvature are technically more difficult to remove.

5. Successful endoscopic resection depends on having histologically clear lateral and vertical margins of the tumor at the time of resection, to be assessed by endoscopic biopsies in follow-up examinations.

6. Assessment of the results of endoscopic resection is based on the rates of complete removal or destruction, en bloc resection, recurrence, and patient survival.

The Japanese Research Society for Gastric Cancer has established the following criteria for lesions suitable for endoscopic resection. Type I or IIa: well differentiated, less than 2 cm, limited to the mucosa, and without histologic ulceration. Type IIc: well differentiated, less than 1 cm, limited to the mucosa, and without ulceration. When these criteria are met the risk of lymph node involvement is only 1.7%.

Experience with endoscopic resection of early gastric cancer has been recorded in various studies. In a retrospective evaluation of 210 patients with early gastric cancer treated with EMR and followed for 15 years, the 5-year survival rate was 86% and the 10-year rate 56%; however, there were no cancer-related deaths.[3] In another study, 106 patients with early gastric cancer up to 2 cm in diameter were treated with complete resection of the lesion in a single procedure, either by en bloc resection for lesions less than 10 mm (64%) or by piecemeal resection for larger lesions (36%); no recurrence after either technique was found in patients with tumor-negative margins, and the overall recurrence rate of cancer was 2.8%.[4] All tumors that recurred were greater than 15 mm initially, and all were treated with piecemeal resection. Histologic reconstruction to confirm complete resection by piecemeal removal often is difficult, therefore patients treated with this method should be followed closely.

Amano and colleagues[5] have retrospectively evaluated endoscopic therapy in patients with early gastric cancer that does not meet the Japanese Research Society morphologic criteria for lesions suitable for EMR. Endoscopic therapy consisted of EMR, thermal therapy, or both. Poorly differentiated and well-differentiated tumors from 1 to 3 cm were included. Some patients with submucosal invasion limited to sm1 also were included. Curative resection is defined as where the lateral and vertical margins of the specimens were free of cancer and there was no submucosal invasion deeper than 500 μm from the muscularis mucosae, lymphatic invasion, or vascular involvement, and it was achieved in 95%. The rate of cure in this group was statistically similar to that of cancers that fulfilled the standard morphologic criteria for EMR resection (98%).[5]

Adequacy of EMR should be assessed by measuring the distance from the margin of the cancer to the edge of the resected specimen. In one study, no cancer recurred when this distance was more than 2 mm, whereas 16% recurred when the distance was less than 2 mm[6]; presence of cancer at the edge of the specimen was associated with a 45.8% recurrence rate. In another study,[7] no recurrence was observed if the distance from the margin of the cancer to the edge of the resected specimen was more than 7 mm. Thus, it seems that adequate distance (preferably at least 2 mm) between the cancer and the edge of the specimen needs to be achieved to ensure a complete resection. Margin-negative resections were more likely (81.2%) in cancers that are less than 1 cm in diameter than in cancers that are more than 2 cm in diameter.[7]

A prospective analysis of 479 early gastric cancers in 405 patients treated with EMR over an 11-year period at Tokyo National Cancer Center has been reported.[8] The selection criteria were as follows: well- or moderately well-differentiated gastric cancer; morphologic type I, IIa, or IIc; no histologic evidence of ulceration; diameter less than 3 cm; histologic confirmation of intramucosal carcinoma; no lymphovascular invasion; and clean margins. Complete resection was achieved in 69% (278 of 405). The recurrence rate was only 2% after complete resection, and all recurrences were treated successfully with a modified combination therapy of EMR and laser. Two hundred seventy-eight lesions were followed after endoscopic treatment for a median period of 38 months (range, 3–120 months); no cancer recurred and no cancer-related deaths were reported.

Recently, EMR and ESD have become established alternatives to surgical therapy for early gastric cancer in Korea and Japan.[9] The traditional indication criteria for endoscopic resection are elevated-type intramucosal cancer (0–IIa) less than 20 mm, depressed-type mucosal cancer without ulceration (0–IIb, 0–IIc) less than 10 mm, and well-differentiated or moderately differentiated intestinal-type adenocarcinoma.

In a report by Abe and colleagues,[10] depressed cancers were associated with lymph node metastases (86%) when there was submucosal infiltration, a size of 20 mm or more, or lymphatic vessel involvement.

Some authors[5,11] have proposed extended indications for EMR in early gastric cancer: well-differentiated lesions up to 30 mm, without an ulcer or ulcer scar; mucosal cancers less than 20 mm, with an ulcer or ulcer scar; sm1 lesions less than 20 mm, without an ulcer or ulcer scar; and poorly differentiated lesions less than 10 mm.

The risk for nodal metastasis for differentiated early or mucosal cancers is approximately 0.4%. Undifferentiated mucosal cancers are not recommended to be treated by EMR, because the higher risk for nodal metastasis is approximately 4%. However, according to one study, poorly differentiated and signet-ring cell carcinomas less than 5 mm in size can be treated with EMR.[12] The proposed extended criteria for endoscopic resection in the ESD era are summarized in **Fig. 1**.

Expansion of the criteria for EMR will reduce the need for gastrectomy in early gastric cancer. However, because resection of large or ulcerated lesions by conventional EMR is difficult, ESD has been developed. Over the years, substantial experience in the use of this technique has been gained. In Japan, ESD performed with the insulation-tip knife or others has become standard treatment of early gastric cancer with estimated minimum metastatic risk.[13–16]

In a report from Europe, ESD was performed with a new double-channel endoscope in 10 patients, nine early gastric cancers and one adenoma with a median diameter of

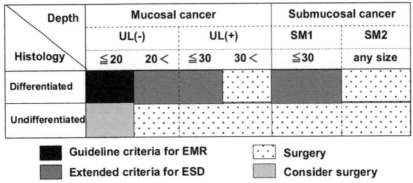

Depth / Histology	Mucosal cancer				Submucosal cancer	
	UL(-)		UL(+)		SM1	SM2
	≤20	20<	≤30	30<	≤30	any size
Differentiated						
Undifferentiated						

■ Guideline criteria for EMR   **⫶** Surgery

■ Extended criteria for ESD   **■** Consider surgery

Fig. 1. Proposed extended criteria for endoscopic resection in the ESD era. SM, submucosal cancer; UL, ulcer.

22 mm (R-scope; Olympus, Tokyo, Japan).[17] ESD was successful in six patients. Perforation occurred in two, who were then treated with surgery.[17] In another study,[18] ESD was performed in 19 patients with superficial gastric lesions (15–30 mm) that had high-grade (N = 15) or low-grade (N = 4) noninvasive epithelial neoplasia. R0 resection was performed in 89% and en bloc resection in 79%. Major bleeding occurred in one patient (5%); there were no perforations. In a median follow-up of 10 months, one cancer (5%) recurred.[18]

Endoscopic resection has been performed also for undifferentiated intramucosal cancer.[19] In 38 such patients with 42 undifferentiated intramucosal cancers, who had declined surgical therapy, ESD was performed with dedicated devices by experienced expert endoscopists. The en bloc resection rate was 83.3% and complete resection rate 80.9%. Clinical remission was achieved in 92.8%, with recurrence in only 7.14%, during follow-up of 15 months. In undifferentiated gastric cancer, grossly normal gastric mucosa surrounding the resected lesion can contain cancer cells beneath the epithelium[20]; this characteristic may explain why the complete resection rate of ESD for undifferentiated cancer is lower than that reported for well-differentiated cancer.

The en bloc resection rate is better with ESD than with conventional EMR. However, the procedure time is longer for ESD, a disadvantage that might be improved with experience.[21-23]

LOWER GASTROINTESTINAL TRACT

Recently, ESD has been increasingly applied to colorectal disease, although it has not become a standard therapeutic procedure for early colorectal carcinoma because of its technical difficulty, the relatively long procedure time required, and the risk of complications, such as perforation and bleeding. Nonetheless, many Japanese endoscopists have reported that, with various new devices,[24-26] colorectal ESD can overcome the technical limitation of EMR and achieve higher en bloc resection rates.[16,27-33] In North America and Europe, the number of medical facilities that perform colorectal ESD has been increasing.[25,34,35]

In Japan, most of the colorectal tumors that are difficult to remove en bloc by EMR are large laterally spreading tumors.[25] When larger than 20 mm in diameter, these tumors are usually removed by piecemeal EMR because of the technical limitation to allow endoscopic resection. Even so, cutting within the adenomatous portion

---

Box 1

Indications for ESD of colorectal tumors according to criteria established by the Colorectal ESD Standardization Implementation Working Group

1. Large (>20 mm in diameter) lesions in which en bloc resection using snare EMR is difficult, although the lesion is otherwise appropriate for endoscopic treatment

   Nongranular, large spreading tumors, particularly those of the pseudodepressed type

   Lesions with type VI pit pattern

   Carcinoma with submucosal infiltration

   Large depressed-type lesions

   Large elevated lesion suspected of being carcinoma[a]

2. Mucosal lesions with fibrosis caused by prolapse from biopsy or peristalsis of the lesions

3. Sporadic localized tumors in the presence of chronic inflammation, such as ulcerative colitis

4. Local residual early carcinoma after endoscopic resection

   [a]Including granular-type laterally spreading tumors and nodular mixed-type tumors.

---

does not affect histologic interpretation of the tissue or curability of the lesion. Granular-type, large spreading tumors containing adenoma or focal cancer in adenoma are acceptable indications for piecemeal EMR, provided the cancerous portion is completely resected en bloc. In such cases, examination of the tumor's pit pattern with magnification chromoendoscopy before attempting piecemeal removal is crucial.[26]

Indications for colorectal ESD recommended by the Colorectal ESD Standardization Implementation Working Group are listed in **Box 1** and summarized as follows[36–38]: (1) lesions difficult to remove en bloc with a snare EMR because of size, such as nongranular large spreading tumors (particularly the pseudodepressed type), lesions with a type Vi pit pattern, and protruding large lesions suspected of being carcinoma; (2) lesions with fibrosis caused by biopsy or from peristalsis; (3) sporadic localized lesions in the presence of chronic inflammation, such as ulcerative colitis; and (4) local residual carcinoma after EMR. ESD for lesions with severe fibrosis is technically difficult.[33] In selecting the best therapy (piecemeal EMR, ESD, or surgical resection) for colonic tumors, it is important to consider not only the features of the lesions, including clinicopathologic aspects and location, but also the local expertise and skill of the colonoscopist, including scope handling, and the predicted duration of the procedure.

Recently, hybrid ESD, which is a combination of ESD and EMR techniques, has been reported useful for resection of small colorectal lesions.[39] Compared with conventional ESD, hybrid ESD requires less time and technical complexity, which are advantages for nonexperts in performing en bloc resection of larger colorectal lesions. Many expert endoscopists advocate that ESD be standard treatment of the removal of large, colorectal neoplasms. To help overcome the learning curve of colorectal ESD, Western and Eastern endoscopic societies should communicate with each other.

REFERENCES

1. Ryu C, Chen Y. Endoscopic therapy for gastric neoplasms. In: Ginsberg G, Gostout C, Kochman M, et al, editors. Clinical gastrointestinal endoscopy. 2nd edition. St Louis (MO): Saunders Elsevier; 2012. p. 425–47.

2. Saito Y, Uraoka T, Yamaguchi Y, et al. A prospective, multicenter study of 1111 colorectal endoscopic submucosal dissections (with video). Gastrointest Endosc 2010;72(6):1217–25.

3. Takekoshi T, Baba Y, Ota H, et al. Endoscopic resection of early gastric carcinoma: results of a retrospective analysis of 308 cases. Endoscopy 1994;26(4):352–8.

4. Tanabe S, Koizumi W, Mitomi H, et al. Clinical outcome of endoscopic aspiration mucosectomy for early stage gastric cancer. Gastrointest Endosc 2002;56(5): 708–13.

5. Amano Y, Ishihara S, Amano K, et al. An assessment of local curability of endoscopic surgery in early gastric cancer without satisfaction of current therapeutic indications. Endoscopy 1998;30(6):548–52.

6. Hamada T, Kondo K, Itagaki Y, et al. Endoscopic mucosal resection for early gastric cancer. Nippon Rinsho 1996;54(5):1292–7 [in Japanese].

7. Mizumoto S, Misumi A, Harada K, et al. Evaluation of endoscopic mucosal resection (EMR) as a curative therapy against early gastric cancer. Nippon Geka Gakkai Zasshi 1992;93(9):1071–4 [in Japanese].

8. Ono H, Kondo H, Gotoda T, et al. Endoscopic mucosal resection for treatment of early gastric cancer. Gut 2001;48(2):225–9.

9. Chung IK, Lee JH, Lee SH, et al. Therapeutic outcomes in 1000 cases of endoscopic submucosal dissection for early gastric neoplasms: Korean ESD Study Group multicenter study. Gastrointest Endosc 2009;69(7):1228–35.

10. Abe N, Watanabe T, Suzuki K, et al. Risk factors predictive of lymph node metastasis in depressed early gastric cancer. Am J Surg 2002;183(2):168–72.

11. Gotoda T. Endoscopic resection for premalignant and malignant lesions of the gastrointestinal tract from the esophagus to the colon. Gastrointest Endosc Clin N Am 2008;18(3):435–50.

12. Makuuchi H, Kise Y, Shimada H, et al. Endoscopic mucosal resection for early gastric cancer. Semin Surg Oncol 1999;17(2):108–16.

13. Gotoda T. A large endoscopic resection by endoscopic submucosal dissection procedure for early gastric cancer. Clin Gastroenterol Hepatol 2005;3(7 Suppl 1): S71–3.

14. Gotoda T, Kondo H, Ono H, et al. A new endoscopic mucosal resection procedure using an insulation-tipped electrosurgical knife for rectal flat lesions: report of two cases. Gastrointest Endosc 1999;50(4):560–3.

15. Kodashima S, Fujishiro M, Yahagi N, et al. Endoscopic submucosal dissection using flexknife. J Clin Gastroenterol 2006;40(5):378–84.

16. Toyonaga T, Man-i M, Chinzei R, et al. Endoscopic treatment for early stage colorectal tumors: the comparison between EMR with small incision, simplified ESD, and ESD using the standard flush knife and the ball tipped flush knife. Acta Chir Iugosl 2010;57(3):41–6.

17. Neuhaus H, Costamagna G, Deviere J, et al. Endoscopic submucosal dissection (ESD) of early neoplastic gastric lesions using a new double-channel endoscope (the "R-scope"). Endoscopy 2006;38(10):1016–23.

18. Dinis-Ribeiro M, Pimentel-Nunes P, Afonso M, et al. European case series of endoscopic submucosal dissection for gastric superficial lesions. Gastrointest Endosc 2009;69(2):350–5.

19. Ryu CB, Kim SG, Jung IS, et al. Is it possible to perform EMR in poorly differentiated type of early gastric cancer? Gastrointest Endosc 2005;61(5):AB238.

20. Kumarasinghe MP, Lim TK, Ooi CJ, et al. Tubule neck dysplasia: precursor lesion of signet ring cell carcinoma and the immunohistochemical profile. Pathology 2006;38(5):468–71.

21. Watanabe K, Ogata S, Kawazoe S, et al. Clinical outcomes of EMR for gastric tumors: historical pilot evaluation between endoscopic submucosal dissection and conventional mucosal resection. Gastrointest Endosc 2006;63(6):776–82.
22. Park YM, Cho E, Kang HY, et al. The effectiveness and safety of endoscopic submucosal dissection compared with endoscopic mucosal resection for early gastric cancer: a systematic review and metaanalysis. Surg Endosc 2011;25(8):2666–77.
23. Lian J, Chen S, Zhang Y, et al. A meta-analysis of endoscopic submucosal dissection and EMR for early gastric cancer. Gastrointest Endosc 2012;76:763–70.
24. Hurlstone DP, Atkinson R, Sanders DS, et al. Achieving R0 resection in the colorectum using endoscopic submucosal dissection. Br J Surg 2007;94(12):1536–42.
25. Kudo S, Lambert R, Allen JI, et al. Nonpolypoid neoplastic lesions of the colorectal mucosa. Gastrointest Endosc 2008;68(Suppl 4):S3–47.
26. Tanaka S, Kaltenbach T, Chayama K, et al. High-magnification colonoscopy (with videos). Gastrointest Endosc 2006;64(4):604–13.
27. Yamamoto H. Endoscopic submucosal dissection of early cancers and large flat adenomas. Clin Gastroenterol Hepatol 2005;3(7 Suppl 1):S74–6.
28. Isomoto H, Nishiyama H, Yamaguchi N, et al. Clinicopathological factors associated with clinical outcomes of endoscopic submucosal dissection for colorectal epithelial neoplasms. Endoscopy 2009;41(8):679–83.
29. Saito Y, Sakamoto T, Fukunaga S, et al. Endoscopic submucosal dissection (ESD) for colorectal tumors. Dig Endosc 2009;21(Suppl 1):S7–12.
30. Hotta K, Oyama T, Shinohara T, et al. Learning curve for endoscopic submucosal dissection of large colorectal tumors. Dig Endosc 2010;22(4):302–6.
31. Niimi K, Fujishiro M, Kodashima S, et al. Long-term outcomes of endoscopic submucosal dissection for colorectal epithelial neoplasms. Endoscopy 2010;42(9):723–9.
32. Yoshida N, Naito Y, Kugai M, et al. Efficient hemostatic method for endoscopic submucosal dissection of colorectal tumors. World J Gastroenterol 2010; 16(33):4180–6.
33. Matsumoto A, Tanaka S, Oba S, et al. Outcome of endoscopic submucosal dissection for colorectal tumors accompanied by fibrosis. Scand J Gastroenterol 2010;45(11):1329–37.
34. Repici A, Hassan C, De Paula Pessoa D, et al. Efficacy and safety of endoscopic submucosal dissection for colorectal neoplasia: a systematic review. Endoscopy 2012;44(2):137–50.
35. Antillon MR, Bartalos CR, Miller ML, et al. En bloc endoscopic submucosal dissection of a 14-cm laterally spreading adenoma of the rectum with involvement to the anal canal: expanding the frontiers of endoscopic surgery (with video). Gastrointest Endosc 2008;67(2):332–7.
36. Tanaka S, Oka S, Kaneko I, et al. Endoscopic submucosal dissection for colorectal neoplasia: possibility of standardization. Gastrointest Endosc 2007;66(1):100–7.
37. Tanaka S, Oka S, Chayama K. Colorectal endoscopic submucosal dissection: present status and future perspective, including its differentiation from endoscopic mucosal resection. J Gastroenterol 2008;43(9):641–51.
38. Tanaka S, Tamegai Y, Tsuda S, et al. Multicenter questionnaire survey on the current situation of colorectal endoscopic submucosal dissection in Japan. Dig Endosc 2010;22(Suppl 1):S2–8.
39. Terasaki M, Tanaka S, Oka S, et al. Clinical outcomes of endoscopic submucosal dissection and endoscopic mucosal resection for laterally spreading tumors larger than 20 mm. J Gastroenterol Hepatol 2012;27(4):734–40.

Expanding Indications for ESD
Submucosal Disease (SMT/Carcinoid Tumors)

Osamu Goto, MD, PhD, Toshio Uraoka, MD, PhD,
Joichiro Horii, MD, PhD, Naohisa Yahagi, MD, PhD*

KEYWORDS

- Submucosal tumor • Carcinoid • Endoscopic submucosal dissection
- Endoscopic full-thickness resection • Laparoscopic-endoscopic cooperative surgery

KEY POINTS

- Endoscopic submucosal dissection (ESD) is useful for submucosal tumors (SMTs) within the superficial submucosal layer, but perforation frequently occurs during ESD for SMTs located at the deeper layer.
- Endoscopic resection for small esophageal SMTs is acceptable, although candidates for endoscopic removal are rare.
- Laparoscopic assistance will be effective for minimally invasive endoscopic local resection for certain types of gastric SMT.
- Endoscopic mucosal resection with a ligation device would be better than ESD for rectal carcinoid in terms of simplicity and effectiveness.

INTRODUCTION—EXPANSION OF INDICATION FOR ESD

Endoscopic submucosal dissection (ESD) has been gaining acceptance worldwide over the past decade due to an enthusiastic introduction by experts as well as clinical evidence showing clinical merits of this technique.[1-4] The prominent advantage of ESD is that gastrointestinal epithelial lesions can be resected endoscopically in an en bloc fashion regardless of size or the existence of scar formation. ESD has allowed patients with early-stage gastrointestinal neoplasms to receive curative resection without possible organ loss. Owing to the minimally invasive nature of endoscopic intervention, surgery has gradually been replaced by this promising technique.

The ESD procedure is composed of the 2 following phases: circumferential mucosal incision and dissection of the connective tissue just below the lesion under direct

Competing Interests: We have no financial relationships relevant to this publication to disclose.
Division of Research and Development for Minimally Invasive Treatment, Cancer Center, School of Medicine, Keio University, 35 Shinanomachi, Shinjuku-ku, Tokyo 160-8582, Japan
* Corresponding author.
E-mail address: yahagi-tky@umin.ac.jp

Gastrointest Endoscopy Clin N Am 24 (2014) 169–181
http://dx.doi.org/10.1016/j.giec.2013.11.006
1052-5157/14/$ – see front matter © 2014 Elsevier Inc. All rights reserved.

visualization. If a resected lesion has a sufficient lateral margin from the circumferential incision and a sufficient vertical margin through subtumoral dissection, complete resection can theoretically be accomplished, implying that ESD can be applied not only to epithelial neoplasms but also to nonepithelial tumors. Indeed, reports of attempts and successes of ESD for submucosal tumors (SMTs) including carcinoid tumors have been increasing over recent years. In this review, the current application of ESD for gastrointestinal tumors other than cancers is summarized, after the characteristics of SMT and carcinoid tumor are reviewed.

SMT

A submucosal tumor is defined as a neoplastic lesion located within the gastrointestinal wall derived from tissue layers other than the epithelium. Representative SMTs are gastrointestinal stromal tumor (GIST), leiomyoma, lipoma, schwannoma, and carcinoid tumor. The incidence of each tumor varies by the organ. Because it is covered with normal epithelium, endoscopic diagnosis is sometimes difficult. Therefore, the term "SMT" can include nonneoplastic lesions as well (eg, cyst, ectopic pancreas). Some epithelial tumors or cancers grow toward the inside of the submucosal layer, which then mimics SMT and can lead to misdiagnosis. There is a consensus that GIST is the most relevant type of SMT. It is thought to be a mesenchymal tumor of mesothelial origin, especially originating from the interstitial cells of Cajal, and it has high likelihood of *c-kit* abnormality. Because it is difficult to distinguish between benign and malignant GIST even by pathologic assessment, GISTs are usually treated as tumors having malignant potential. In clinical settings, a treatment strategy is decided based on the risk of aggressive behavior of the tumor.[5,6]

Endoscopic ultrasonography (EUS) is indispensable for accurate preoperative diagnosis. EUS offers various information about the tumor (ie, the size, location, shape, and echogenicity). Therefore, an extramural compression or cyst, mimicking an SMT, can be excluded from SMT that needs to be treated.[7–9] Nevertheless, it is still difficult to distinguish GIST from other mesenchymal tumors (leiomyoma or schwannoma). When EUS shows a hypoechoic, well-demarcated SMT derived from the muscularis mucosa or the mucularis propria, endoscopic ultrasound-guided fine-needle aspiration is recommended to obtain histologic diagnosis.[10–12]

In terms of treatment, a potentially malignant SMT (ie, GIST) would be a candidate for resection. Principally, any resection technique would be acceptable if en bloc resection is achieved, but endoscopic local resection is more preferable because of its minimally invasive nature. In the "pre-ESD" era, however, endoscopic en bloc local resection of SMT was technically challenging with relatively higher risk of complications. These procedures were done only by some endoscopists in the manner of modified endoscopic mucosal resection (EMR) to obtain histologic assessment of the tumor.[13,14] Through the emergence of ESD, the possibility of en bloc resection increased, even for SMTs.[15–25] Accordingly, ESD has been applied to SMT nowadays, although highly advanced endoscopic skills are required.

CARCINOID TUMOR

Carcinoid tumors, one of the neuroendocrine tumors, are most frequently found in the gastrointestinal tract, especially in the appendix and the small intestine. It arises from a deeper layer in the mucosa and easily invades the submucosa, rupturing the muscularis mucosa. Growth of this tumor is generally indolent, but it is treated as a potentially malignant tumor. Indeed, angiolymphatic infiltration or metastasis to distant organs often occurs as it progresses.

In clinical settings, small carcinoids located in the rectum, the duodenum, or the stomach would be good candidates for endoscopic resection, especially EMR. There is a certain amount of consensus that endoscopic resection in the rectum is acceptable for a carcinoid 10 mm or less in size that is confined within the submucosal layer because of a low likelihood of metastasis.[26,27] On the other hand, gastric carcinoids are divided into 4 categories according to the clinicopathological features[28]: type 1, arising multifocally in patients with autoimmune gastritis; type 2, arising multifocally in patients with multiple endocrine neoplasia type 1; type 3, arising sporadically and solely in patients without underlying diseases; and type 4, poorly differentiated neuroendocrine carcinomas, arising solely and growing aggressively. Because small carcinoids except for type 4 show indolent growth, endoscopic resection is recommended as the first choice for histologic investigation. Similarly to other neoplasms, complete resection without angiolymphatic invasion is essential to achieve curative resection.[28]

ESD FOR ESOPHAGEAL SUBMUCOSAL TUMOR

Prevalence of SMTs in the esophagus is relatively low compared with the stomach. In most cases, esophageal SMTs are found incidentally, small and often only intermittently symptomatic, and may be considered as a candidate for endoscopic removal. In esophageal SMTs, leiomyoma and granular cell tumors are frequently seen, followed by GISTs, whereas carcinoids are quite rare. Because the number of esophageal SMTs is small and the clinicopathological behavior is still largely unknown, no established consensus regarding the treatment of esophageal SMTs exists. Therefore, the indication of treatment mainly depends on the decision at each institution as well as the patient's preference. Several studies have shown the feasibility of endoscopic resection of esophageal SMTs, and that the optimal size for the resection is suggested to be 1 to 2 cm,[15–17,29–32] considering the durability of transoral retrieval and the possibility of postoperative stricture (**Table 1**).

From the viewpoint of the principle of ESD, endoscopic removal is easier and safer in esophageal SMTs limited to the submucosal layer than located in the muscularis propria or deeper (**Fig. 1**). Esophageal SMTs within the submucosal layer can be resected using conventional ESD technique, although endoscopists should be aware that the dissecting layer is thinner than that for epithelial lesions. On the other hand, ESD for SMT arising from the muscularis propria has a high possibility of perforation. Accordingly, preoperative assessment for the depth of SMT by EUS is mandatory for estimation of the origin of tumor and thus for the risk of ESD, as Shim and Jung[33] have proposed that treatment strategy should be primarily determined by the depth of the lesion.

Table 1
Outcomes of endoscopic resection for esophageal submucosal tumor

Authors/Reference No./Year	Target	Average Size (cm)	Method	N	Complete Resection (%)	Perforation (%)
Chiu et al,[15] 2006	SMT	1.0	ESD	1	100	0
Shi et al,[16] 2011	SMT-MP	1.3	ESD	30	93.3	6.7
Liu et al,[17] 2012	SMT-MP	2.1	ESD	14	92.9	7.1
Gong et al,[30] 2012	SMT-MP	1.7	ESTD	8	100	0
Inoue et al,[31] 2012	SMT	1.5	ESTD	3	100	0
Ye et al,[32] 2013	SMT	1.8	ESTD	15	100	20

Abbreviations: ESTD, endoscopic submucosal tunneling dissection; MP, arising from muscularis propria.

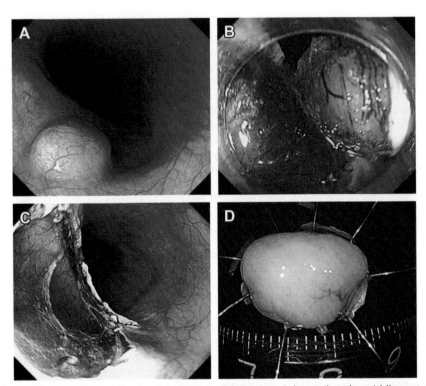

Fig. 1. ESD for esophageal submucosal tumor. (*A*) A tumor is located at the middle part of the esophagus 12 mm in diameter. (*B*) The tumor lifted well by submucosal injection is supposed to be confined within the submucosal layer. (*C*) The submucosal layer beneath the lesion is clearly visualized. (*D*) The tumor is resected in one piece without damage to the tumor surface.

Park and colleagues[34] demonstrated the feasibility of endoscopic enucleation with an insulated-tip knife with the purpose of curative resection as well as precise histologic assessment. One drawback, however, was that complete resection by histologic assessment may be difficult due to a burning effect on the surface of the tumor because the mucosa just above the lesion has to be cut longitudinally. In this regard, ESD would be simpler than the reported technique because the area that should be dissected is limited to the plane just below the tumor, which may be the reason the number of reports about the feasibility of ESD is larger than that of endoscopic enucleation.[15–17,29]

As technical skills of ESD advance, ESD for esophageal SMTs arising from the muscularis propria has been reported.[16,17,30] The perforation rate was relatively high (a maximum of 12.9%) compared with conventional ESD, but in most cases, it could be well treated endoscopically by clipping. Due to the invasiveness of surgery, ESD for esophageal SMTs at the deeper layers can be considered for one of the treatment modalities if secure endoscopic maneuverability and methods would be assured.

One concern that should be taken into consideration in esophageal ESD for SMT is postoperative stricture. Endoscopic enucleation by submucosal tunneling is a newly invented technique that prevents postresection stricture by preserving the covering mucosa of the SMT.[30–32] Because the mucosa and the muscularis mucosae remain, the esophageal lumen can stay free of stricture. This concept was derived from per-oral endoscopic myotomy for achalasia.[35] In per-oral endoscopic myotomy, the circular muscle bundles under the submucosal tunnel are cut longitudinally to dilate the esophageal lumen. Because the muscularis mucosa is untouched, stenosis of the lumen can be avoided. Endoscopic enucleation using the submucosal tunneling technique also requires highly advanced endoscopic skill but is promising as a less-invasive endoscopic surgery if the target lesion is small enough (less than approximately 3 cm) to retrieve through the submucosal tunnel.[31]

ESD FOR GASTRIC SUBMUCOSAL TUMOR

Gastric SMTs are not rare, and they are estimated to increase in accordance with increased use of esophagogastroduodenoscopy and improvement of diagnostic modalities. GISTs are most common among SMTs of the stomach and also are frequently considered for resection. Laparoscopic or open surgery is regarded as the standard approach; however, endoscopic resection also became available and is considered feasible for smaller lesions after establishment of ESD technique.

In the similar way of the history of development in ESD, various attempts at endoscopic removal of SMTs in gastrointestinal tract have been started from the resection of gastric submucosal lesions. Lee and colleagues[18] reported the feasibility of ESD in 12 gastric SMTs arising from muscularis propria without perforation, although the complete resection rate was not very high (75%). They also suggested that EMR using the cap method was helpful for remnant SMTs after ESD. However, en bloc resection is still desirable for accurate histologic analysis as well as the purpose of curative resection. For SMTs arising from the muscularis propria especially, en bloc resection may lead to perforation. Some reports have shown the safety of ESD for SMTs with sacrificed complete resection rate, whereas other reports revealed feasibility of complete resection by ESD with a risk of complication (**Table 2**).[18–22]

There are 2 approaches to solve this dilemma. One approach is ESD combined with laparoscopic assistance. Hiki and colleagues[38] developed laparoscopic and endoscopic cooperative surgery (LECS), which comprises 3 steps: endoscopic circumferential mucosal incision using the ESD technique, endoscopic or laparoscopic circumferential seromuscular incision after endoscopic intentional perforation, and laparoscopic suturing. This method allows the resection area to be as small as

Table 2
Outcomes of endoscopic resection for gastric submucosal tumor

Authors/Reference No./Year	Target	Average Size (cm)	Method	N	Complete Resection (%)	Perforation (%)
Lee et al,[18] 2006	SMT-MP	2.1	ESD	12	75	0
Hoteya et al,[19] 2009	SMT-MM	3.8	ESD	9	100	0
Bialek et al,[20] 2012	SMT	2.5[a]	ESD	37	81.1	5.4
Li et al,[21] 2012	SMT-MP at EGJ	1.8	ESD	143	94.4	4.2
Zhang et al,[22] 2012	SMT-MP at EGJ	1.6	ESD	68	95.6	10.3
Zhou et al,[36] 2011	SMT	2.8	EFTR	26	100	—
Schlag et al,[37] 2013	SMT	1.5	EFTR	14	100	—

Abbreviations: EFTR, endoscopic full-thickness resection; EGJ, esophagogastric junction; MM, arising from muscularis mucosa; MP, arising from muscularis propria.
[a] Median.

possible, which can prevent postoperative complications such as dumping syndrome or the stagnation of food. Other local resection techniques for endoscopy and laparoscopy have been introduced as modified natural orifice translumenal endoscopic surgery procedures.[39,40] Furthermore, nonexposed endoscopic wall-inversion surgery (NEWS) has been developed as an alternative method to LECS.[41] The ESD technique is also used in NEWS: first, laparoscopic circumferential seromuscular incision after endoscopic submucosal fluid injection; second, laparoscopic seromuscular suture tucking the inverted lesion into the inside of the stomach; third, endoscopic circumferential incision for inverted protrusion using the ESD technique. This technique enables minimally sized gastric local resection without transluminal communication, which would cause neither contamination nor tumor seeding into the abdominal space. Therefore, NEWS would be also a minimally invasive surgical option for gastric cancer, simply by combining it with laparoscopic lymph node dissection.

The other concept for endoscopic resection of SMTs is ESD with iatrogenic perforation followed by closure (see **Table 2**). Defined literally, endoscopic resection with intentional perforation is called endoscopic full-thickness resection (EFTR),[36,37,42] and endoscopic resection without intentional perforation (but with high rate of perforation for SMT) is called ESD.[18–22,29] Although perforation has to be avoided as much as possible, perforation during the latter approach can be resolved by endoscopic treatment (**Fig. 2**). Zhou and colleagues[36] demonstrated the feasibility of EFTR in a

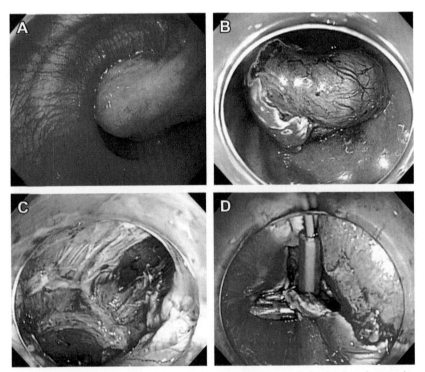

Fig. 2. ESD for esophagogastric junctional tumor. (*A*) A tumor is located at the esophagogastric junction 23 mm in diameter. (*B*) The tumor was mostly dissected but part of the tumor was attached to the proper muscle layer. (*C*) The tumor was completely resected but partial muscle defect was observed. (*D*) The muscle defect was completely closed with loop snare and endo-clips.

case series, and Wang and colleagues[29] elucidated the usefulness of ESD compared with laparoscopic resection in a comparative study. Both EFTR and ESD for gastric SMTs showed successful results, but a secure closure method should still be necessary in order for these techniques to be accepted as a general approach. Although endoscopic enucleation was also reported,[43] the same problem for secure closure should be solved. However, endoscopic enucleation with submucosal tunneling may not require endoscopic closure of defect if the tunnel is long enough to interrupt transluminal communication.[30,31,44]

Generally, the laparoscopic approach mentioned above is necessary for larger tumors, such as SMTs measuring 3 cm or more in diameter, because transoral retrieval is difficult. Transarterial embolization before EFTR might be effective to downsize the volume of tumor,[45] although whole histologic assessment becomes impossible. Further investigation is necessary for this approach.

Solitary small gastric carcinoids are also an indication for endoscopic resection.[46] Although sufficient evidence is still lacking, endoscopic resection is technically simple. Because a target lesion is small, EMR with other methods (aspiration with a cap, a ligation device, grasping forceps) may be comparable to, or possibly more suitable than, ESD.

ESD FOR COLORECTAL SUBMUCOSAL TUMOR

Unlike the upper gastrointestinal tract, typical SMTs are not so common in the colorectum. In nonepithelial tumors, rectal carcinoids are most frequently seen as candidates for endoscopic resection. Endoscopic resection of rectal tumors can be a great benefit to patients in terms of organ preservation, especially anal function. Therefore, safe and secure endoscopic resection for rectal carcinoid tumor has been widely investigated and accepted as a primary modality for small carcinoid tumors.

Small carcinoid tumors (10 mm or less) located within the submucosa would be an indication for endoscopic resection (**Table 3**). Published data show favorable results of ESD for rectal carcinoid tumors.[23–25,51–55] High rates of complete resection (80%–100%) compared with conventional endoscopic resection (50%–80%) and low complication rates (less than 5%) reflect the technical advantages of ESD for rectal carcinoid tumors. Because tumor size is relatively small, and most lesions are located within the superficial layer in the rectum, ESD may be easily accepted with less difficulty. Interestingly, earlier published reports tend to demonstrate the feasibility of ESD in comparison with EMR,[23–25,52] whereas some later articles showed the equality or superiority of EMR to ESD.[47–50] Conventional EMR is inferior to ESD regarding the completeness of resection, whereas EMR with a ligation device (EMR-L) may be superior to ESD in terms of procedural period or hospitalization period. It is interesting that EMR-L has been reevaluated for rectal carcinoids in recent years, when ESD tends to be the so-called last resort (**Fig. 3**).

Colorectal ESD for SMTs (except for carcinoid tumors) is rarely reported.[56] There may be 2 major reasons: the prevalence of colorectal SMTs that should be treated is low, and the merit of organ preservation in the colon cannot outweigh the demerit of ESD (eg, extremely high risk for perforation, need for highly advanced skill, time-consuming procedure). Unlike the esophagus or the stomach, local resection of the colon is less likely to cause a loss of quality of life after surgery. If laparoscopic resection is selected, recovery course and morbidity after surgery are generally acceptable with low mortality. As a result, indication of ESD for colorectal SMTs seems quite limited.

Table 3
Comparative studies of endoscopic resection for rectal carcinoid

Authors/Reference No./Year	Method	N	Average Size (mm)	Complete Resection (%)	Perforation (%)	Conclusion
Zhou et al,[23] 2010	ESD, EMR	20, 23	7.2, 6.7	100, 52.2	5, 0	ESD > EMR
Park et al,[24] 2010	ESD, EMR	31, 62	6.5, 7.1	90.3, 71.0	3.2, 1.6	ESD > EMR
Lee et al,[25] 2010	ESD, EMR	46, 28	6.2, 5.7	82.6, 64.3	2.2, 0	ESD > EMR
Zhao et al,[47] 2012	EMR-C, EMR, ESD	10, 10, 10	—	100, 80, 100	0, 0, 0	EMR-C > EMR, ESD
Niimi et al,[48] 2012	EMR-L, ESD	11, 13	4.4, 5.5	100, 92.3	0, 0	EMR-L > ESD
Kim et al,[49] 2012	EMR-L, EMR, ESD	40, 31, 44	4.0, 4.8, 4.3	100, 77.4, 97.7	2.5, 0, 0	EMR-L, ESD > EMR
Choi et al,[50] 2013	EMR-L, ESD	29, 31	4.3, 5.2	82.8, 80.6	0, 0	EMR-L > ESD

Abbreviations: C, with capping technique; L, with ligation technique.

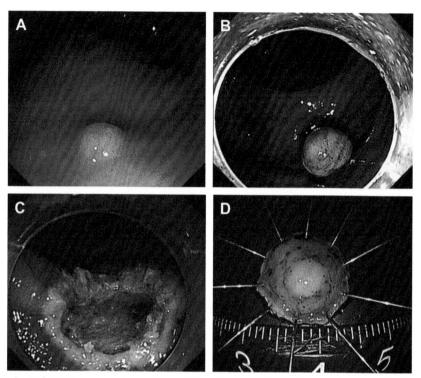

Fig. 3. Endoscopic mucosal resection with a ligation device for rectal carcinoid. (*A*) A yellowish tumor 5 mm in diameter is covered with the normal epithelium. (*B*) The tumor is protruded by ligation with an O-ring after submucosal injection. (*C*) The lesion is removed using a snare hanging below the ring. (*D*) En bloc resection is completed easily in a short time.

ESD FOR SUBMUCOSAL TUMOR IN OTHER ORGANS

Theoretically speaking, ESD for duodenal lesions would be ideal in terms of less invasiveness and organ preservation, especially because pancreaticoduodenectomy is one of the most invasive surgeries and other treatment modalities should be selected as much as possible as appropriate. Endoscopic resection, however, is also quite difficult and risky for several reasons: poor maneuverability of the endoscope, very thin wall of duodenum, existence of bile and pancreatic juice, and so on. Nevertheless, ESD for duodenal carcinoids might be acceptable with highly experienced hands because of the advantage of the location,[57] although it is surely controversial.[46] In the current situation, laparoscopy-assisted local resection such as LECS would be the best choice as endoscopic resection for duodenal SMT.[58] However, there is some risk for intraperitoneal tumor dissemination in performing LECS by which transluminal communication is unavoidable. Therefore, only SMTs without ulcer formation should be considered for this technique.

FUTURE PERSPECTIVES

Irrespective of the organ, there remains plenty of unknown information, including the natural course of SMTs. Concretely defined indication of ESD for SMT is also yet to be established. To acquire further information, resection as a complete biopsy should be warranted. From this point of view, ESD for SMT would be acceptable with discussed merits of ESD if the safety of the procedure can be assured by reliable endoscopic skills and local expertise. Further investigation, including long-term outcomes, is required to establish ESD as a primary treatment of SMT.

ACKNOWLEDGMENTS

We thank Motoki Sasaki (Cancer Center, Keio University School of Medicine) for collecting the endoscopic images.

REFERENCES

1. Ono H, Kondo H, Gotoda T, et al. Endoscopic mucosal resection for treatment of early gastric cancer. Gut 2001;48:225–9.
2. Yamamoto H, Kawata H, Sunada K, et al. Successful en-bloc resection of large superficial tumors in the stomach and colon using sodium hyaluronate and small-caliber-tip transparent hood. Endoscopy 2003;35:690–4.
3. Oyama T, Tomori A, Hotta K, et al. Endoscopic submucosal dissection of early esophageal cancer. Clin Gastroenterol Hepatol 2005;3:S67–70.
4. Yahagi N, Uraoka T, Ida Y, et al. Endoscopic submucosal dissection using the Flex and the Dual knives. Tech Gastrointest Endosc 2011;13:74–8.
5. Fletcher CD, Bermann JJ, Corless C, et al. Diagnosis of gastrointestinal stromal tumors: a consensus approach. Hum Pathol 2002;33:459–65.
6. Miettinen M, Lasota J. Gastrointestinal stromal tumors: pathology and prognosis at different site. Semin Diagn Pathol 2006;23:70–83.
7. Rösch T, Kapfer B, Will U, et al. Accuracy of endoscopic ultrasonography in upper gastrointestinal submucosal lesions: a prospective multicenter study. Scand J Gastroenterol 2002;7:856–62.
8. Oztas E, Oguz D, Kurt M, et al. Endosonographic evaluation of patients with suspected extraluminal compression or subepithelial lesions during upper gastrointestinal endoscopy. Eur J Gatroenterol Hepatol 2011;23:586–92.
9. Goto O, Kambe H, Niimi K, et al. Discrepancy in diagnosis of gastric submucosal tumor among esophagogastroduodenoscopy, CT, and endoscopic ultrasonography: a retrospective analysis of 93 consecutive cases. Abdom Imaging 2012;37:1074–8.
10. Hoda KM, Rodriguez SA, Faigel DO, et al. EUS-guided sampling of suspected GI stromal tumors. Gastrointest Endosc 2009;69:1218–23.
11. Sepe PS, Moparty B, Pitman MB, et al. EUS-guided FNA for the diagnosis of GI stromal cell tumors: sensitivity and cytologic yield. Gastrointest Endosc 2009;70:254–61.
12. Mekky MA, Yamao K, Sawaki A, et al. Diagnostic utility of EUS-guided FNA in patients with gastric submucosal tumors. Gastrointest Endosc 2010;71:913–9.
13. Yoshikane H, Suzuki T, Yoshioka N, et al. Duodenal carcinoid tumor: endosonographic imaging and endoscopic resection. Am J Gastroenterol 1995;90:642–4.
14. Kajiyama T, Hajiro K, Sakai M, et al. Endoscopic resection of gastrointestinal submucosal lesions: a comparison between strip biopsy and aspiration lumpectomy. Gastrointest Endosc 1996;44:404–10.
15. Chiu PW, Lee YT, Ng EK. Resection of esophageal leiomyoma using an endoscopic submucosal dissection technique. Endoscopy 2006;38(Suppl 2):E4.

16. Shi Q, Zhong YS, Yao LQ, et al. Endoscopic submucosal dissection for treatment of esophageal submucosal tumors originating from the muscularis propria layer. Gastrointest Endosc 2011;74:1194–200.

17. Liu BR, Song JT, Qu B, et al. Endoscopic muscularis dissection for upper gastrointestinal subepithelial tumors originating from the muscularis propria. Surg Endosc 2012;26:3141–8.

18. Lee IL, Lin PY, Tung SY, et al. Endoscopic submucosal dissection for the treatment of intraluminal gastric subepithelial tumors originating from the muscularis propria layer. Endoscopy 2006;38:1024–8.

19. Hoteya S, Iizuka T, Kikuchi D, et al. Endoscopic submucosal dissection for gastric submucosal tumor, endoscopic sub-tumoral dissection. Dig Endosc 2009;21:266–9.

20. Białek A, Wiechowska-Kozłowska A, Pertkiewicz J, et al. Endoscopic submucosal dissection for treatment of gastric subepithelial tumors (with video). Gastrointest Endosc 2012;75:276–86.

21. Li QL, Yao LQ, Zhou PH, et al. Submucosal tumors of the esophagogastric junction originating from the muscularis propria layer: a large study of endoscopic submucosal dissection (with video). Gastrointest Endosc 2012;75:1153–8.

22. Zhang Y, Ye LP, Zhu LH, et al. Endoscopic muscularis excavation for subepithelial tumors of the esophagogastric junction originating from the muscularis propria layer. Dig Dis Sci 2012;58:1335–40.

23. Zhou PH, Yao LQ, Qin XY, et al. Advantages of endoscopic submucosal dissection with needle-knife over endoscopic mucosal resection for small rectal carcinoid tumors: a retrospective study. Surg Endosc 2010;24:2607–12.

24. Park HW, Byeon JS, Park YS, et al. Endoscopic submucosal dissection for treatment of rectal carcinoid tumors. Gastrointest Endosc 2010;72:143–9.

25. Lee DS, Jeon SW, Park SY, et al. The feasibility of endoscopic submucosal dissection for rectal carcinoid tumors: comparison with endoscopic mucosal resection. Endoscopy 2010;42:647–51.

26. Scherübl H. Rectal carcinoids are on the rise: early detection by screening endoscopy. Endoscopy 2009;41:162–5.

27. Park CH, Cheon JH, Kim JO, et al. Criteria for decision making after endoscopic resection of well-differentiated rectal carcinoids with regard to potential lymphatic spread. Endoscopy 2011;43:790–5.

28. Scherübl H, Cadiot G, Jensen RT. Neuroendocrine tumors of the stomach (gastric carcinoids) are on the rise: small tumors, small problems? Endoscopy 2010;42:664–71.

29. Wang L, Fan CQ, Ren W, et al. Endoscopic dissection of large endogenous myogenic tumors in the esophagus and stomach is safe and feasible: a report of 42 cases. Scand J Gastroenterol 2011;46:627–33.

30. Gong W, Xiong Y, Zhi F, et al. Preliminary experience of endoscopic submucosal tunnel dissection for upper gastrointestinal submucosal tumors. Endoscopy 2012;44:231–5.

31. Inoue H, Ikeda H, Hosoya T, et al. Submucosal endoscopic tumor resection for subepithelial tumors in the esophagus and cardia. Endoscopy 2012;44:225–30.

32. Ye LP, Zhang Y, Mao XL, et al. Submucosal tunnelling endoscopic resection for the treatment of esophageal submucosal tumours originating from the muscularis propria layer: an analysis of 15 cases. Dig Liver Dis 2013;45:119–23.

33. Shim CS, Jung IS. Endoscopic removal of submucosal tumors: preprocedure diagnosis, technical options, and results. Endoscopy 2005;37:646–54.

34. Park YS, Park SW, Kim TI, et al. Endoscopic enucleation of upper-GI submucosal tumors by using an insulated-tip electrosurgical knife. Gastrointest Endosc 2004;59:409–15.
35. Inoue H, Minami H, Kobayashi Y, et al. Peroral endoscopic myotomy (POEM) for esophageal achalasia. Endoscopy 2010;42:265–71.
36. Zhou PH, Yao LQ, Qin XY, et al. Endoscopic full-thickness resection without laparoscopic assistance for gastric submucosal tumors originated from the muscularis propria. Surg Endosc 2011;25:2926–31.
37. Schlag C, Wilhelm D, von Delius S, et al. EndoResect study: endoscopic full-thickness resection of gastric subepithelial tumors. Endoscopy 2013;45:4–11.
38. Hiki N, Yamamoto Y, Fukunaga T, et al. Laparoscopic and endoscopic cooperative surgery for gastrointestinal stromal tumor dissection. Surg Endosc 2008; 22:1729–35.
39. Abe N, Takeuchi H, Yanagida O, et al. Endoscopic full-thickness resection with laparoscopic assistance as hybrid NOTES for gastric submucosal tumor. Surg Endosc 2009;23:1908–13.
40. Nakajima K, Nishida T, Takahashi T, et al. Partial gastrectomy using natural orifice translumenal endoscopic surgery (NOTES) for gastric submucosal tumors: early experience in humans. Surg Endosc 2009;23:2650–5.
41. Goto O, Mitsui T, Fujishiro M, et al. New method of endoscopic full-thickness resection: a pilot study of non-exposed endoscopic wall-inversion surgery in an ex vivo porcine model. Gastric Cancer 2011;14:183–7.
42. Ikeda K, Fritscher-Ravens A, Mosse CA, et al. Endoscopic full-thickness resection with sutured closure in a porcine model. Gastrointest Endosc 2005;62: 122–9.
43. Chu YY, Lien JM, Tsai MH, et al. Modified endoscopic submucosal dissection with enucleation for treatment of gastric subepithelial tumors originating from the muscularis propria layer. BMC Gastroenterol 2012;12:124.
44. Sumiyama K, Gostout CJ, Rajan E, et al. Submucosal endoscopy with mucosal flap safety valve. Gastrointest Endosc 2007;65:688–94.
45. Chikamori F, Kuniyoshi N, Okamoto H, et al. A case of a gastric submucosal tumor treated with combined therapy using superselective TAE and endoscopic local resection. Surg Laparosc Endosc Percutan Tech 2012;22:e297–300.
46. Suzuki S, Ishii N, Uemura M, et al. Endoscopic submucosal dissection (ESD) for gastrointestinal carcinoid tumors. Surg Endosc 2012;26:759–63.
47. Zhao ZF, Zhang N, Ma SR, et al. A comparative study on endoscopy treatment in rectal carcinoid tumors. Surg Laparosc Endosc Percutan Tech 2012;22:260–3.
48. Niimi K, Goto O, Fujishiro M, et al. Endoscopic mucosal resection with a ligation device or endoscopic submucosal dissection for rectal carcinoid tumors: an analysis of 24 consecutive cases. Dig Endosc 2012;24:443–7.
49. Kim KM, Eo SJ, Shim SG, et al. Treatment outcomes according to endoscopic treatment modalities for rectal carcinoid tumors. Clin Res Hepatol Gastroenterol 2012;37:275–82.
50. Choi CW, Kang DH, Kim HW, et al. Comparison of endoscopic resection therapies for rectal carcinoid tumor: endoscopic submucosal dissection versus endoscopic mucosal resection using band ligation. J Clin Gastroenterol 2013; 47:432–6.
51. Yamaguchi N, Isomoto H, Nishiyama H, et al. Endoscopic submucosal dissection for rectal carcinoid tumors. Surg Endosc 2010;24:504–8.
52. Onozato Y, Kakizaki S, Iizuka H, et al. Endoscopic treatment of rectal carcinoid tumors. Dis Colon Rectum 2010;53:169–76.

53. Moon SH, Hwang JH, Sohn DK, et al. Endoscopic submucosal dissection for rectal neuroendocrine (carcinoid) tumors. J Laparoendosc Adv Surg Tech A 2011;21:695–9.
54. Hamada Y, Tanaka K, Tano S, et al. Usefulness of endoscopic submucosal dissection for the treatment of rectal carcinoid tumors. Eur J Gastroenterol Hepatol 2012;24:770–4.
55. Sung HY, Kim SW, Kang WK, et al. Long-term prognosis of an endoscopically treated rectal neuroendocrine tumor: 10-year experience in a single institution. Eur J Gastroenterol Hepatol 2012;24:978–83.
56. Konuma H, Fu K, Konuma I, et al. A rectal GI stromal tumor completely resected with endoscopic submucosal dissection (with video). Gastrointest Endosc 2011; 73:1322–5.
57. Matsumoto S, Miyatani H, Yoshida Y. Endoscopic submucosal dissection for duodenal tumors: a single-center experience. Endoscopy 2013;45:136–7.
58. Kato M, Nakajima K, Nishida T, et al. Local resection by combined laparoendoscopic surgery for duodenal gastrointestinal stromal tumor. Diagn Ther Endosc 2011;2011:1–7.

Electrocautery for ESD
Settings of the Electrical Surgical Unit VIO300D

Yoshinori Morita, MD, PhD

KEYWORDS

- Endoscopic submucosal dissection • Electrosurgical unit • VIO300D
- Power peak system

KEY POINTS

- An electrical surgical unit (ESU) is an apparatus for performing incisions and coagulation through applying Joule heat, generated by a high-frequency current (high-frequency alternating current: 300 kHz to 5 MHz), onto tissue without neuromuscular stimulation.
- Output by the ESU includes incision output and coagulation output. Incision output is needed to generate a steam explosion (spark) by quickly raising the intracellular fluid temperature through continuous application of Joule heat generated by the high-frequency current (unmodulated pulse: continuous wave).
- To perform safe and successful endoscopic submucosal dissection, one must fully understand the principles and features of an ESU to use settings that match the device and to adjust the settings appropriately for each situation.

 A case presentation of electrocautery for ESD accompanies this article

INTRODUCTION

The rapid advancement of endoscopic treatment for gastrointestinal tumors that has occurred recently has quickly transformed the era of traditional polypectomy and endoscopic mucosal resection into the era of endoscopic submucosal dissection (ESD).[1–5] Accordingly, to perform safe and effective treatment while minimizing complications, one must fully understand the principles and features of the electrosurgical units (ESUs) that are used for ESD, and choose the appropriate, case-dependent settings for each surgical instrument, depending on the equipment, lesions, and organs.

This article describes the optimal settings for the ESU VIO300D (ERBE Elektromedizin GmbH, Tubingen, Germany) (**Fig. 1**), and how its features can be fully used for safe and effective ESD.

Department of Gastroenterology, Kobe University School of Medicine, 7-5-1, Kusunoki-cho, Chuo-ku, Kobe 650-0017, Japan
E-mail address: ymorita@med.kobe-u.ac.jp

Gastrointest Endoscopy Clin N Am 24 (2014) 183–189
http://dx.doi.org/10.1016/j.giec.2013.11.008
1052-5157/14/$ – see front matter © 2014 Elsevier Inc. All rights reserved.

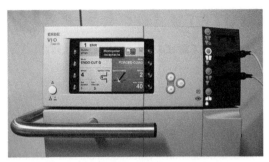

Fig. 1. VIO300D (ERBE Elektromedizin GmbH, Tubingen, Germany).

ESU DESCRIPTION

An ESU is an apparatus for performing incisions and coagulation through applying Joule heat, generated by a high-frequency current (high-frequency alternating current: 300 kHz to 5 MHz), onto tissue without neuromuscular stimulation. The higher the current density is (ie, more current per unit of area), the greater the Joule heat. To incise tissue requires a steam explosion (spark). During incision, electrical resistance is continually changing, depending on many factors, such as the shape of the surgical instrument, contact area, movement speed, and the electrical conductivity of the target tissue. Therefore, with the conventional ESU, which is an output control type, the incision and depth of coagulation is not constant because of changes in voltage that accompany changes in resistance.

The solution to this problem is a voltage-control type of ESU, which is based on the principle that the discharge distance (coagulation depth) is proportional to the voltage. Thus, by sensing the voltage between the active electrode and the tissue in real time through an internal high-speed sensor circuit and continuing to maintain the correct voltage setting through instantaneous feedback, consistent incision and coagulation depth can be maintained with high reproducibility. In particular, using this voltage-control type of ESU for ESD, which demands precision, is recommended.

DIFFERENCES BETWEEN CUT OUTPUT AND COAGULATION OUTPUT

Output of the ESU includes incision output and coagulation output, as described earlier. Incision output is needed to generate a steam explosion (spark) by quickly raising the intracellular fluid temperature through continuous application of Joule heat generated by the high-frequency current (unmodulated pulse: continuous wave). On the other hand, coagulation output is applied to dehydrate and dry tissue by slowly raising the intracellular and extracellular fluid temperature through intermittently applying Joule heat (modulated pulse: intermittent wave). ESUs are known to act differently above and below a borderline of 200 peak voltage (Vp). Because a spark is generated when more than 200 Vp is applied, an incision effect can be created even from the coagulation output when the current density is high and the contact area is narrow. This effect is dependent on the status of the current density at the tip of the device and the surface area of tissue contact. That is, ESD can be performed using coagulation output because the requirements are fulfilled. Conversely, only dehydration and drying of the tissue occur without spark generation when the voltage is less than 200 Vp, even with continuous wave; this is called *SOFT COAG mode*, and it plays an important role in contact coagulation when treating vessels for hemostasis during management and prevention of bleeding in ESD. Therefore, the waveform, such as continuous or intermittent, is selected only for the pace of Joule heat generation.

FEATURES OF VIO300D

VIO300D is an evolutionary outcome of the conventional intelligent cut and coagulation (ICC) series. The main features are as follows:

1. Conventional ENDO CUT has improved and evolved to ENDO CUT I and Q.
2. DRY CUT and SWIFT COAG, new incision, and dissection output settings are provided for ESD.
3. The power peak system (PPS) works on all cut outputs (see next section).
4. The amount of current is doubled and the amount of heat generated is improved 4-fold compared with the ICC 200 series.
5. Voltage control or arc control is possible for all cut/coagulation outputs.

The basic output philosophy of the VIO300D is an unmodulated (continuous wave) or pulse-modulated sine wave (burst wave) with the frequency of 350 kHz, regardless of whether it is for incision or coagulation. In other words, the waveform that repeats the amplitude 350,000 times per second (continuous wave) or the intermittent waveform using only a few percent of amplitude that repeats 350,000 times (burst wave) is applied for incision and coagulation. The belief is that a large difference can result in incision and coagulation depth when the Vp is different, and that there can be differences in incision and coagulation ability when the duty cycle is different because of pulse modulation, even if the frequency and conduction time are the same.

NEW FEATURES OF THE VIO300D

The VIO300D's various functions are optimal for ESD. New features developed from the ICC series are described.

DRY CUT and SWIFT COAG

Although the output wave of the DRY CUT and SWIFT COAG is the pulse-modulated sine wave (burst wave), it allows both incision and coagulation through changes in the duty cycle (**Fig. 2**). In other words, the duty cycle is less than 10% in FORCED COAG, which is the basis of the coagulation wave, but is 30% in DRY CUT and 20% in SWIFT COAG.

DRY CUT has a higher amount of current per cycle compared with SWIFT COAG so that its incision ability is superior. Conversely, SWIFT COAG has a higher voltage than DRY CUT, and therefore its hemostatic ability is higher. In addition, the PPS function works for DRY CUT so that a smooth incision is possible with less hemorrhaging without catching at incision initiation or with any time lag. The PPS is the function that assists incision by releasing the upper limit of output to allow instantaneous flow of the maximum current of 4 A within 200 W when high output is needed, such as the moment of incision initiation.

ENDO CUT I and Q

The ENDO CUT mode of the ICC 200 alternates automatically between SOFT COAG (750 ms) and HIGH CUT (50 ms) to make an incision after vessels are coagulated by SOFT COAG (**Fig. 3**).[6] This mode is a breakthrough, and has allowed tissue to incised with less bleeding. For the ENDO CUT mode of the ICC 200 series, the coagulation depth is controlled through changing the Vp (Effect), and output (W) was defined as the instantaneous workload. In other words, when Effect is increased, the incision

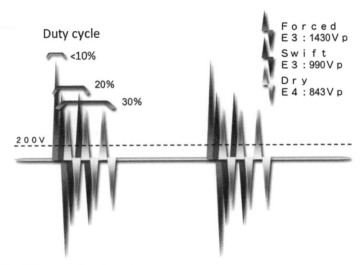

Fig. 2. The difference of each mode.

and coagulation abilities are increased proportionally and simultaneously. Therefore, the ICC 200 could not handle the situation that requires reduction of the coagulation depth while maintaining only the incision ability. However, in the newer model (VIO300D), Vp is fixed (550 and 770 V for ENDO CUT I and Q, respectively), and instead of fine-tuning by output (W), 3 parameters (hemostatic effect: Effect; width of incision: cut duration; and speed of incision: cut interval) can be selected individually so that the desired output corresponding to each situation can be produced. In other words, the setting is possible in the range of Effect 1 through 4 (0–400 Vp), cut duration 1 through 4 (I: 8–32 ms, Q: 2–14 ms), and cut interval 1 through 10 (400–1840 ms). For example, only the coagulation effect can be changed at the time of incision without changing the incision effect through optionally setting the voltage during the incision with Effect. Separately, the width of a single incision and the speed of incision can be adjusted by the cut duration and cut interval, respectively.

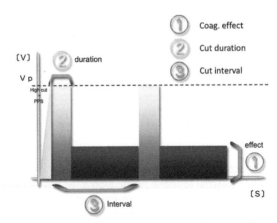

Fig. 3. ENDO CUT mode of the VIO300D. Coag., coagulation; Coag. effect, coagulation effect; PPS, power peak system; Vp, peak voltage.

SPECIFIC SETTINGS IN THE ENDOSCOPY UNIT FOR VIO300D

To perform safe and successful ESD, one must fully understand the principles and features of an ESU to use settings that match the device and to adjust the settings appropriately for each situation. To perform ESD in the authors' hospital, the insulation-tipped (IT) knife (KD-610L, Olympus Optical Co, Ltd, Tokyo, Japan) or IT-2 knife (KD-611L, Olympus) is used (**Fig. 4**) for gastric tumors,[7] and the Flush Knife (DK-2618JN, FUJIFILM Optical Co, Ltd, Tokyo, Japan) or Flush Knife BT (DK-2618JB, FUJIFILM) (**Fig. 5**) is used for esophageal and colorectal tumors.[8–11] However, it is considered important and effective to use a needle-type device (ie, Flush Knife/Flush Knife BT) in addition to the IT knives (ie, IT and IT-2 knives) for gastric tumors if significant submucosal fibrosis is present, such as from gastric ulcer scars. Because the contact area of the tip of the needle-type knife is smaller than that of the IT knife, the current density is greater and the incision ability is improved, thereby increasing perforation occurrence. Also, with the high incision ability, the cutting movement speed of the knife tip is more likely to increase, and therefore the coagulation depth would be shallower and bleeding would be more likely. Therefore, when using a needle-type device, it is desirable to attain the coagulation effect when the pinpoint incision or dissection is performed intentionally at a slower pace while applying minimal tension. In this maneuver, tactical skills of the operator are demanded, such as maneuvering the scope and working the pedal to control the discharge of the ESU. Because the walls of the esophagus and colon are thinner than those of the stomach, fine-tuning is necessary to control the coagulation depth to a required and sufficient degree by using ENDO CUT I (Vp: 550 V) with reduced Effect. The different settings for each device in the authors' hospital are shown in **Table 1**; however, these settings tend to differ at various institutions.

CASE PRESENTATION

A bundle of large penetrating vessels in the submucosa was found during ESD for a lateral spreading tumor granular-type of the rectum (Video 1). After vessels were fully

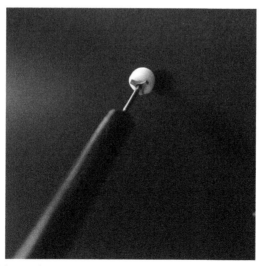

Fig. 4. IT-2 knife (Olympus).

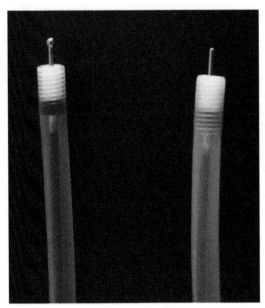

Fig. 5. Flush Knife and Flush Knife BT (FUJIFILM).

Table 1
The settings used for each device at Kobe University

Esophagus	Flush Knife BT 1.5 mm				
Marking	SOFT COAG	E5	100 W		
Mucosal incision	ENDOCUT I	E4 D3 I3			
Submucosal dissection	FORCED COAG	E2	50 W		
	SWIFT COAG	E2	50 W		
Hemostasis (Coagrasper)	SOFT COAG	E5	100 W		

Stomach	Flush Knife BT 2.5 mm			IT knife 2	
Marking	SOFT COAG	E5	100 W	APC 2	Forced APC, E1, 30 W, 1.0 L/min
Mucosal incision	ENDOCUT I	E2 D3 I2		ENDO CUT I (precut)	E4 D2 I3
				ENDO CUT Q	E2 D3 I2
Submucosal dissection	FORCED COAG	E3	50 W	FORCED COAG E3	100 W
	SWIFT COAG	E3	50 W	SWIFT COAG E3	100 W
Hemostasis (Coagrasper)	SOFT COAG	E5	100 W	SOFT COAG E5	100 W

Colorectum	Flush Knife BT 1.5 mm				
(Marking)	SOFT COAG	E5	100 W		
Mucosal incision	ENDOCUT I	E2 D3 I3			
Submucosal dissection	FORCED COAG	E2	50 W		
	SWIFT COAG	E2	50 W		
Hemostasis (Coagrasper)	SOFT COAG	E5	100 W		

exposed by Flush Knife BT with FORCED COAG, coagulation was performed with the Coagrasper forceps (FD-410LR for upper GI or FD-410QR for lower GI, Olympus) using SOFT COAG to dehydrate and seal up the vessel. Submucosal dissection was then completed successfully with the SWIFT COAG mode.

SUPPLEMENTARY DATA

Video related to this article can be found online at http://dx.doi.org/10.1016/j.giec.2013.11.008.

REFERENCES

1. Ono H, Kondo H, Gotoda T, et al. Endoscopic mucosal resection for treatment of early gastric cancer. Gut 2001;48:225–9.
2. Rosch T, Sarbia M, Schumacher B, et al. Attempted endoscopic en bloc resection of mucosal and submucosal tumors using insulated-tip knives: a pilot series. Endoscopy 2004;36:788–801.
3. Yamamoto H, Yahagi N, Oyama T. Mucosectomy in the colon with endoscopic submucosal dissection. Endoscopy 2005;37:764–8.
4. Oda I, Gotoda T, Hamanaka H, et al. Endoscopic submucosal dissection for early gastric cancer: technical feasibility, operation time and complications from a large consecutive series. Dig Endosc 2005;17:54–8.
5. Neuhaus H, Costamagna G, Deviere J, et al. Endoscopic submucosal dissection of early gastric lesions using a new double channel endoscope (the "R-scope"). Endoscopy 2006;38:1016–23.
6. Kohler A, Maier M, Benz C, et al. A new HF current generator with automatically controlled system (Endocut mode) for endoscopic sphincterotomy-preliminary experience. Endoscopy 1998;30:351–5.
7. Ono H, Hasuike N, Inui T, et al. Usefulness of a novel electrosurgical knife, the insulation-tipped diathermic knife-2, for endoscopic submucosal dissection of early gastric cancer. Gastric Cancer 2008;11:47–52.
8. Toyonaga T, Nishino E, Hirooka T, et al. Use of short needle knife for esophageal endoscopic submucosal dissection. Dig Endosc 2005;17:246–52.
9. Toyonaga T, Nishino E, Hirooka T, et al. Intraoperative bleeding in endoscopic submucosal dissection in the stomach and strategy for prevention and treatment. Dig Endosc 2006;18:S123–7.
10. Toyonaga T, Nishino E, Dozaiku T, et al. Management to prevent bleeding during endoscopic submucosal dissection using the flush knife for gastric tumors. Dig Endosc 2007;19:S14–8.
11. Toyonaga T, Man-I M, Fujita T, et al. The performance of a novel ball-tipped Flush knife for endoscopic submucosal dissection: a case-control study. Aliment Pharmacol Ther 2010;32:908–15.

Endoscopic Submucosal Dissection (ESD) Versus Simplified/Hybrid ESD

Takashi Toyonaga, MD[a,b,*], Mariko Man-I, MD, PhD[b], Yoshinori Morita, MD, PhD[b], Takeshi Azuma, MD, PhD[b]

KEYWORDS

- ESD • Colon • Rectum • Simplified ESD • Hybrid ESD

KEY POINTS

- Endoscopic submucosal dissection (ESD) with snaring (simplified or hybrid ESD) is a good option for filling the gap between conventional endoscopic mucosal resection and full ESD.
- ESD with snaring is considered a good introductory step to ESD.
- The simplification of ESD through the development of new devices and modified methods is still required because ESD is often the best treatment for early stage colorectal tumors.

INTRODUCTION

Endoscopic submucosal dissection (ESD) theoretically enables en bloc resection regardless of size and shape; however, it has pitfalls such as the technical difficulty, long procedure time, and high frequency of perforation.[1–5] In the colorectum, the lumen is narrow, it bends, and the wall is thin; therefore, the risk of complication is much higher than in the stomach. The use of ESD in the colorectum should be carefully considered.

With endoscopic mucosal resection (EMR), used in cases in which the size of the lesion is larger than 2 cm, the rate of piecemeal resection increases significantly. However, even if a lesion is smaller than 2 cm, it may be difficult to remove by EMR because of the location and/or the existence of nonlifting signs. The most difficult locations are the backside of folds, the corners, and the areas neighboring diverticulum.

[a] Department of Endoscopy, Kobe University Hospital, Kobe, Hyogo 650-0019, Japan; [b] Frontier Medical Science in Gastroenterology, Kobe University School of Medicine, Kobe, Hyogo 650-0019, Japan
* Corresponding author. Department of Endoscopy, Kobe University Hospital, 7-5-1 Kusumoki, Chuo, Kobe, Hyogo, Japan.
E-mail address: toyonaga@med.kobe-u.ac.jp

Gastrointest Endoscopy Clin N Am 24 (2014) 191–199
http://dx.doi.org/10.1016/j.giec.2013.11.004
1052-5157/14/$ – see front matter © 2014 Elsevier Inc. All rights reserved.

Nonlifting signs are a result of either severe fibrosis or massive invasion into the submucosal layer.

Colorectal tumors that can be treated by endoscopic resection vary greatly from small sessile and 0–IIc type lesions to huge lateral spreading tumors that occupy almost the whole round of the rectum. The treatment methods of colorectal lesions also diverge into many branches, including hot biopsy, polypectomy, EMR, and

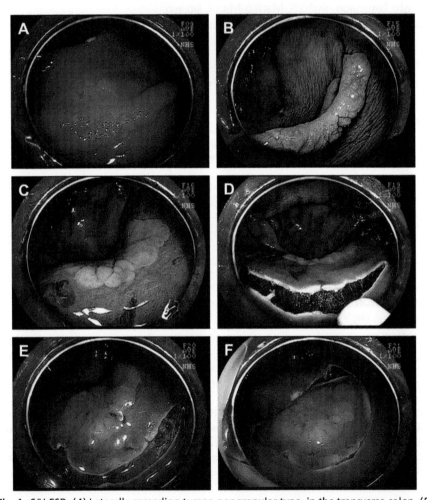

Fig. 1. S/H-ESD. (*A*) Laterally spreading tumor, nongranular type, in the transverse colon. (*B*) Chromoendoscopy (indigo carmine) shows clear border of the lesion, which spread widely over the fold. (*C*) The lesion was lifted up by injection sodium hyaluronate in to the submucosal layer. (*D*) Mucosal incision by using a ball-tipped Flush knife. (*E*) The view after 2/3 circumferential mucosal incision. The lesion is sifting up to the oral side by the tension of the remaining mucosa. (*F*) Condition after completion of circumferential incision and some amount of submucosal dissection. The groove around the lesion was successfully created. (*G*) The view on snaring. The snaring was easily performed by fixing the snare along the submucosal groove. (*H*) Condition after the resection. Procedure time was 25 minutes. (*I*) The resected specimen. Specimen size was 35 × 25 mm and tumor size was 22 × 17 mm. Histopathological finding reveled intramucosal cancer. Resection margin was free.

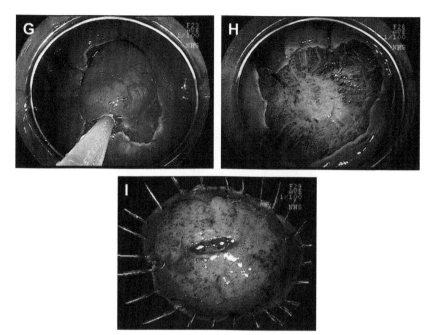

Fig. 1. (*continued*)

ESD. In the colorectum, detailed preoperative diagnoses with magnified observation clearly show whether lesions must be removed by en bloc resection or require piece-meal resection. It is important to choose the proper treatment method for each lesion, taking the clinicopathological background and technical aspects into account, as well as the resources that are needed to make EMR more reliable and ESD easier, safer, and quicker. To fill the gap between conventional EMR and full ESD, ESD with snaring, termed simplified or hybrid ESD (S/H-ESD) was proposed. This article compares the performance of S/H-ESD with full ESD.

METHODS

S/H-ESD is shown in **Fig. 1**. Lesions were resected by snaring after circumferential incision and submucosal dissection to a certain degree.[6–8] Sodium hyaluronate was used for the local injection solution. The tip of snare, Flex knife (Olympus Co, Tokyo, Japan), and Flush knife (Fujifilm Co, Tokyo, Japan) were used for the mucosal incision. This method was considered a good adaptation for lesions that were less than 3 to 4 cm. In cases in which snaring was difficult even after some amount of submucosal dissection, full ESD was attempted. The cases were classified as S/H-ESD when snaring was planned from the beginning and as ESD when snaring was only performed after a trial of full ESD.

ESD is shown in **Fig. 2**. As described in previous reports,[9–13] Flex and Flush knives were used as endoknives. Needle knives, ST hoods, and hook knives were used together depending on the situation. The cases resected by ESD included those in which the treatment method had shifted from S/H-ESD and the recurrent cases after EMR.

These methods were adapted step-by-step. When conventional EMR was too diffi-cult, S/H-ESD was tried first and ESD was tried next.

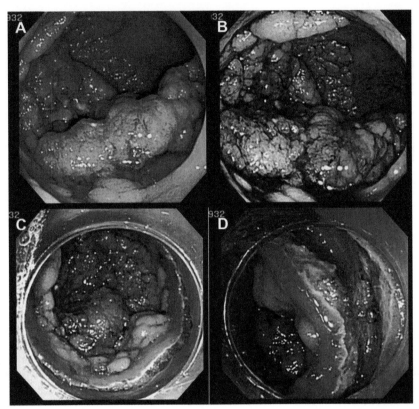

Fig. 2. ESD. (*A, B*) Laterally spreading tumor-granular, nodular mixed type, in the rectum. The lesion occupied 5/6 circumference. (*C*) Condition after semi-circumferential mucosal incision. (*D*) Branch vessels were dissected and some amount of submucosal dissection was performed. Mucosal flap was successfully created. (*E*) The view during the submucosal dissection. Large penetrating vessels were clearly observed. (*F*) Condition after resection. Procedure time was 140 minutes. (*G*) The resected specimen. Specimen size was 112 × 80 mm and tumor size was 105 × 75 mm. Histopathological finding reveled intramucosal cancer in adenoma. Resection margin was free. Oral side is indicated by the *arrow*.

CLINICAL RESULTS

The authors treated 44 colorectal tumors using S/H-ESD and 468 colorectal tumors using ESD. S/H-ESD was performed only by the first author. ESD was performed by two experienced endoscopists (T.T. and Y.M.), including the first author, and by three endoscopists supervised by the authors (T.T. and Y.M.). Tumor sizes, resected specimen sizes, procedure times, en bloc resection rates, and complication (perforation and delayed bleeding) rates were compared between S/H-ESD and ESD. Values are expressed as medians. Statistical analysis was performed using the Fisher test and the Mann-Whitney U-test. A *P* value of less than or equal to 0.05 was considered significant.

Table 1 shows the results of these methods and characteristics of the lesions. The median tumor size was 17 mm (range 4–33) in S/H-ESD and 30 mm (range 6–158) in ESD (S/H-ESD vs ESD, *P*<.0001). The median resected specimen size was 26 mm

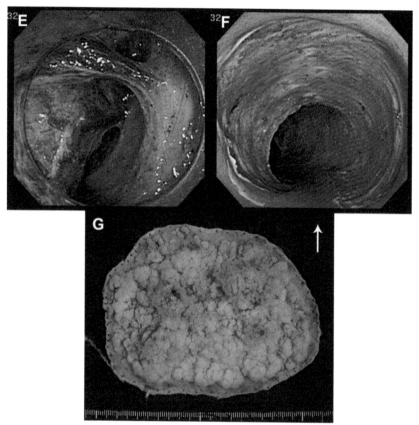

Fig. 2. *(continued)*

(range 13–45) in S/H-ESD and 41 mm (range 17–165) in ESD (S/H-ESD vs ESD, $P<.0001$). The procedure time was 27 minutes (range 8–98) in S/H-ESD and 60 minutes (range 11–335) in ESD (S/H-ESD vs ESD, $P<.0001$). The en bloc resection rate was 90.9% in S/H-ESD and 98.9% in ESD. The en bloc resection rate of ESD was significantly higher than that of S/H-ESD (S/H-ESD vs ESD, $P = .0044$). The complication (delayed bleeding, perforation) rate was 2.3%, 4.5% in S/H-ESD, and 1.5%, 1.5% in ESD (S/H-ESD vs ESD, $P = $ nonsignificant). The complication rate in S/H-ESD tended to be higher than that in the ESD group.

DISCUSSION

There is no clear definition of S/H-ESD. When an endoscopist attempts snaring after circumferential mucosal incision and some amount of submucosal dissection using an ESD device such as the Flush knife, the method tends to be termed S/H-ESD. Hirao and colleagues[14] originally reported on endoscopic resection with local injection of hypertonic saline epinephrine (ERHSE). However, at that time, any amount of submucosal dissection was performed and no specialized devices could be used. Technical difficulty and the risk of complication were higher than that of EMR; therefore, ERHSE did not become widely used.

Table 1
Characteristics of lesions and results

		S/H-ESD	ESD
Lesions		44	468
Median tumor size (mm), range		17 (4–33) [a]	30 (6–158)
Median specimen size (mm), range		26 (13–45) [b]	41 (17–165)
Median procedure time (min), range		27 (8–98) [c]	60 (11–335)
En bloc resection rate (%)		90.9 (40/44) [d]	98.9 (463/468)
Perforation (%)		4.5 (2/44) [e]	1.5 (7/468)
Delayed bleeding (%)		2.3 (1/44) [f]	1.5 (7/468)
Wall invasion (%)	Adenoma	22 (50.0)	161 (34.4)
	Mucosal cancer	17 (38.6)	227 (48.5)
	Submucosal cancer	5 (11.4)	78 (16.7)
	Muscularis propria invasive cancer	0 (0.0)	2 (0.4)

[a] $P<.0001$.
[b] $P<.0001$.
[c] $P<.0001$.
[d] $P = .0044$.
[e] P = nonsignificant.
[f] P = nonsignificant.

Filling the gap between conventional EMR and full ESD is a common aspiration among endoscopists. S/H-ESD, by using ESD devices and snares, is thought to be a candidate for making EMR more reliable and for making ESD easier, safer, and quicker. Thus, the usefulness of S/H-ESD should be examined.

The treatment results of ESD surpassed S/H-ESD and the frequency of perforation and delayed bleeding of S/H-ESD was not significantly lower than that of ESD. Other investigators reported similar results (**Table 2**).[2,3] Endoscopists should note that S/H-ESD was not safer than ESD.

These facts suggest that ESD could be the gold standard for lesions that require reliable en bloc resection. However, there are colorectal lesions that can be fully cured by piecemeal resection[15,16] and there are lesions smaller than 3 to 4 cm that are often not suitable for ESD due to the difficulty getting into the submucosal layer. S/H-ESD is expected to get better results than conventional EMR if it is adapted to these lesions. Moreover, it seems that S/H-ESD is a good introduction to ESD. On the other hand, endoscopic treatments are not the sole treatment modality. Laparoscopic surgery may be a good choice for colonic lesions because the functional disturbance after surgical treatment is thought to be no different than that after endoscopic treatment.[17,18] However, in cases in which the lesions are located in the rectum, the functional disturbance can become a problem after surgical treatment. ESD is suggested to be the best treatment method for early-stage rectal tumors, even if the tumors extend into the anal canal.

Table 2
Outcomes of S/H-ESD and ESD

Author	Method	Lesions	Tumor Size (mm), (range)	Procedure Time (minutes), (range)	En Bloc Resection (%)	Perforation (%)	Delayed Bleeding (%)
Yoshida et al,[7] 2013	S/H-ESD	22	21.2 (10–40)	57 (18–85)	77.3	4.5	4.5
	ESD	466	31.2 (12–130)	94 (10–420)	92.2	3.8	2.5
Oka et al,[8] 2013	S/H-ESD	36	(20–NR)	NR	100	5.6	NR
	ESD	95	(20–NR)	NR	NR	1.1	NR
Toyonaga et al,[6] 2009	S/H-ESD	44	17 (4–33)	27 (8–98)	90.9	4.5	2.3
	ESD	468	30 (6–158)	60 (11–335)	98.9	1.5	1.5

Abbreviation: NR, not reported.

SUMMARY

ESD with snaring (S/H-ESD) is a good option for filling the gap between conventional EMR and full ESD and is considered a good introductory step to ESD. On the other hand, the simplification of ESD through the development of new devices and modified methods is still required because ESD can be the best treatment method for early stage colorectal tumors.

REFERENCES

1. Fujishiro M, Yahagi N, Kakushima N, et al. Outcomes of endoscopic submucosal dissection for colorectal epithelial neoplasms in 200 consecutive cases. Clin Gastroenterol Hepatol 2007;6:678–83.
2. Tanaka S, Oka S, Kaneko I, et al. Endoscopic submucosal dissection for colorectal neoplasia: possibility of standardization. Gastrointest Endosc 2007;66: 100–7.
3. Taku K, Sano Y, Fu KI, et al. Iatrogenic perforation associated with therapeutic colonoscopy: a multicenter study in Japan. J Gastroenterol Hepatol 2007;22: 1409–14.
4. Tanaka S, Oka S, Chayama K. Colorectal endoscopic submucosal dissection: present status and future prospective, including its differentiation from endoscopic mucosal resection. J Gastroenterol 2008;43:641–51.
5. Toyonaga T, Man-I M, Ivanov D, et al. The results and limitations of endoscopic submucosal dissection for colorectal tumors. Acta Chir Iugosl 2008; 55:17–23.
6. Toyonaga T, Man-I M, Morita Y, et al. The new resources of treatment for early stage colorectal tumors: EMR with small incision and simplified endoscopic submucosal dissection. Dig Endosc 2009;21:S31–7.
7. Yoshida N, Yagi N, Naito Y. Hybrid ESD techniques for colorectal tumor ESD. Intestine 2013;17:51–8 [in Japanese with English abstract].
8. Oka S, Tanaka S, Terasaki M, et al. Hybrid ESD for colorectal tumors. Stom Intest 2013;48:185–92 [in Japanese with English abstract].
9. Toyonaga T, Man-I M, Fujita T, et al. Retrospective study for technical aspects and complications of endoscopic submucosal dissection for laterally spreading tumors of the colorectum. Endoscopy 2010;42:714–22.
10. Toyonaga T, Man-I M, Fujita T, et al. The performance of a novel ball-tipped Flush knife for endoscopic submucosal dissection: a case-control study. Aliment Pharmacol Ther 2010;32:908–15.
11. Toyonaga T, Man-I M, Fujita T, et al. Endoscopic submucosal dissection using the Flush knife and the Flush knife BT. Tech Gastrointest Endosc 2011;13:84–90.
12. Toyonaga T, Nishino E, Man-I M, et al. Principles of quality controlled endoscopic submucosal dissection with appropriate dissection level and high quality resected specimen. Clin Endosc 2012;45:362–74.
13. Toyonaga T, Man-I M, East JE, et al. 1,635 Endoscopic submucosal dissection cases in the esophagus, stomach and colorectum: complication rates and long-term outcomes. Surg Endosc 2013;27:1000–8.
14. Hirao M, Masuda K, Asanuma T, et al. Endoscopic resection with local injection of hypertonic saline epinephrine. Gastrointest Endosc 1983;34:264–9.
15. Uraoka T, Saito Y, Matsuda T, et al. Endoscopic indications for endoscopic mucosal resection of laterally spreading tumors in the colorectum. Gut 2006; 55:1592–7.

16. Hurlstone DP, Sanders DS, Cross SS, et al. Colonoscopic resection of lateral spreading tumours: a prospective analysis of endoscopic mucosal resection. Gut 2004;53:1334–9.
17. Weeks JC, Nelson H, Gelber S, et al. Short-term quality-life outcomes following laparoscopic-assisted colectomy vs open colectomy for colon cancer: a randomized trial. JAMA 2002;287:321–8.
18. Jayne DF, Gluillou PG, Thorpe H, et al. Randomized trial of laparoscopic-assisted resection of colorectal carciinoma; 3-year results of the UK MRC CLASSIC Trial group. J Clin Oncol 2007;25:3061–8.

Esophageal ESD
Technique and Prevention of Complications

Tsuneo Oyama, MD, PhD

KEYWORDS

- Endoscopic submucosal dissection (ESD) • Esophageal ESD • Endoscopic clip
- Perforation

KEY POINTS

- The advantage of endoscopic submucosal dissection (ESD) is the ability to achieve high R0 resection, providing low local recurrence rate.
- Esophageal ESD is technically more difficult than gastric ESD due to the narrower space of the esophagus for endoscopic maneuvers.
- Also, the risk of perforation is higher because of the thin muscle layer of the esophageal wall. Blind dissection should be avoided to prevent perforation.
- A clip with line method is useful to keep a good endoscopic view with countertraction.
- Only an operator who has adequate skill should perform esophageal ESD.

INTRODUCTION

Esophageal endoscopic mucosal resection (EMR) was developed in the late 1980s, and it quickly became widely accepted as the treatment of superficial esophageal cancers.[1–4] There was limitation in resectable size, however, and precise resection was impossible. Piecemeal resection was performed for larger lesions, but local recurrence after piecemeal EMR was high.[5] Therefore, a novel endoscopic treatment, ESD, was developed to resolve such disadvantages of EMR.[6–10]

Ten years have passed since esophageal ESD was established. Now, much newer equipment has been developed to make esophageal ESD safer and easier.

ENDOKNIVES

Many endoknives have been developed for ESD. The basic knives are the Hook Knife (KD-620LR, Olympus, Tokyo, Japan) and the Dual Knife (KD-650, Olympus). The insulated tip (IT) knife is widely used for gastric ESD but is not suitable for esophageal ESD, because of a higher perforation rate. Recently, however, the ITknife nano (KD-612, Olympus) was developed for colonic and esophageal ESD.

Department of Gastroenterology, Saku Central Hospital, 197 Usuda, Saku, Nagano 3840301, Japan
E-mail address: oyama@coral.ocn.ne.jp

Gastrointest Endoscopy Clin N Am 24 (2014) 201–212
http://dx.doi.org/10.1016/j.giec.2013.12.001
1052-5157/14/$ – see front matter © 2014 Elsevier Inc. All rights reserved.

The size of the insulation tip is smaller than that of the usual IT knife, and good maneuverability in narrow space is now obtainable. The FlushKnife (Fujifilm, Tokyo, Japan) is a unique new device that incorporates a water flush function. It is useful for additional injection during submucosal dissection. Recently, scissor-like knives, such as the Clutch Cutter (Fujifilm) and the SB Knife (Sumitomo Bakelite, Tokyo, Japan), have been developed. Their cutting speed is slow, but they are easy for beginners to use.

MARKING

The lateral extension of squamous cell carcinoma can be diagnosed easily after 0.75% to 1% iodine dye spray chromoendoscopy. Marks should be placed 2 or 3 mm away from the edge of the unstained area that represents the cancer. The esophageal wall is thinner than that of stomach; therefore, perforation can occur during marking if a needle knife is used. Hook and Dual Knives are useful devices to place the marks safely. The tips of both knives can be retracted within the sheath, and a sharp mark can be placed when the tip of knife is contacted with the mucosa and coagulated by soft coagulation (effect 4, 20 W) (**Fig. 1**).

SUBMUCOSAL INJECTION

Glycerol (Chugai Pharmaceutical, Tokyo, Japan) is injected into the submucosal layer to separate the mucosa from the proper muscular layer. This solution includes 10% glycerin and 0.9% NaCl. Its viscosity is higher than that of saline, and the mucosal elevation could be maintained for longer duration.

MUCOSAL INCISION

The strategy for making a mucosal incision depends on the type of endoknife. When a Dual Knife or Hook Knife is used, the mucosal incision is performed from the oral side. At first, the backside of the Hook Knife is contacted with the mucosa, and a hole is made by endocut I mode (effect 3) (**Fig. 2**). After that, the tip of the Hook Knife is

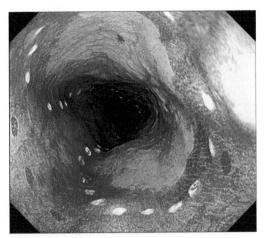

Fig. 1. The tip of the hook knife can be retracted within the sheath, and a sharp mark can be placed when the tip of the Hook Knife makes contact with the mucosa. The author uses soft coagulation (effect 4, 20 W).

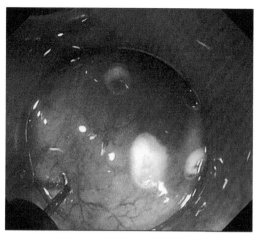

Fig. 2. The author initially places the backside of the Hook Knife in contact with the mucosa after submuosal injection and then makes a mucosal defect using the endocut I mode.

inserted into the submucosal layer, and the mucosa is hooked and cut with the hook part of the knife (**Fig. 3**). This is an important part of the process in order to prevent perforation. The arm part of the Hook Knife is used for longitudinal mucosal incision. The direction of the Hook Knife is turned to the esophageal lumen, and the knife is inserted into the submucosal layer by sliding the backside. Then, the mucosa is captured by the arm part of the knife (**Fig. 4**), and, finally, the mucosa is cut by the combination of spray coagulation (effect 2, 60 W) and endocut mode (effect 3, duration 2, and interval 2). It is an important part of the procedure in order to prevent bleeding during mucosal incision. The submucosal vessels cannot always be observed by endoscopy. Sometimes they are cut unexpectedly, and bleeding occurs during mucosal incision. The initial spray coagulation can coagulate submucosal vessel; therefore, such unexpected bleeding can be prevented with initial spray coagulation.

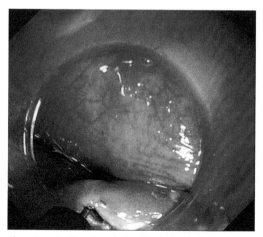

Fig. 3. Next, the author inserts the tip of the Hook Knife into the submucosal layer and hooks and cuts the mucosa with the hook part of the knife.

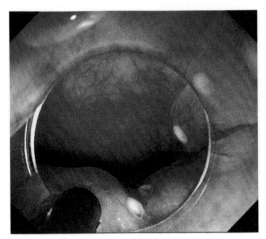

Fig. 4. The arm part of the Hook Knife is used for longitudinal mucosal incision. The author directs the Hook Knife to the lumen and inserts it into the submucosal layer by sliding the back of the knife. Then the mucosa is elevated to the lumen by the arm part of the knife. Finally, the author cuts the mucosa.

A deeper cut of submucosal fibers is performed after mucosal incision. The Hook Knife is inserted into the submucosal layer, and submucosal fibers are hooked and cut. The lesion then shrinks by the contraction of muscularis mucosa (**Fig. 5**). After that, the mucosal incision and deeper cut of the other side is performed and a circumferential incision is completed. When an IT nanoknife is used, the mucosal incision should be started from the anal side. The initial mucosal incision of the anal side is made by a needle knife at first after submucosal injection. After that, the mucosal incision is made by IT nanoknife by endocut mode. The operator cannot see the next mark well, because the cutting direction is always from distal to proximal. Therefore, the operator should take care to avoid cutting inside of the marks.

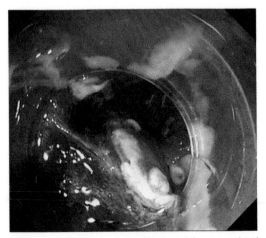

Fig. 5. The Hook Knife is inserted into the submucosal layer, and submucosal fibers are hooked and cut.

SUBMUCOSAL DISSECTION

The direction of gravity should be checked before submucosal dissection is started. Submucosal dissection should be started from the lower side, because water and blood flow to the lower side causes the field of vision to become worse. Therefore, the operator should try to shift the lesion to the upper side. If submucosal dissection is begun from the upper side, the resected part shifts to the lower side, and submucosal dissection of the later half becomes difficult.

A Tunneling Method

Tunnel-like dissection is necessary for circumferential ESD.[11] At first, a circumferential mucosal incision of anal and oral part is performed (**Fig. 6**). After that, a mucosal tunnel is made from oral to anal (**Fig. 7**),[11] and the second tunnel is made at the opposite side. Finally, the remaining submucosal fibers are dissected between the 2 tunnels (**Fig. 7C**).

Clip with Line Methods

If the target lesion can be pulled, good countertraction can be made. The author and colleagues[12] reported on a clip with line method in 2002 (**Fig. 8**). It is a simple and useful method for using countertraction during ESD. A long, 3-0 silk line is tied to the arm part of the clip (HX-610-135, Olympus) (**Fig. 9**). Then the clip with line is reset in the cassette. The scope is withdrawn when the circumferential incision is finished. A clip applicator device (HX-110QR, Olympus) is inserted into the accessory channel of the endoscope, and the clip with line is mounted onto the tip of the applicator. The scope is inserted again, and the submucosal side of the target lesion is grasped (**Fig. 10**). After that, the line is pulled gently. Only a small amount of tension is required to create countertraction. This method also creates a clear field of vision (**Fig. 11**). During submucosal dissection, tension is maintained with a 10-g weight, such as a bite block mouthpiece, attached to the line. The 10-g weight creates sufficient countertraction and tension without threatening to tear the submucosal layer.[13]

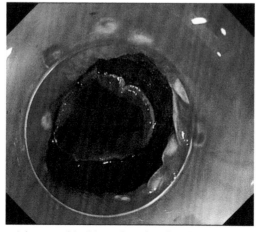

Fig. 6. A circumferential mucosal incision of anal and oral part was performed.

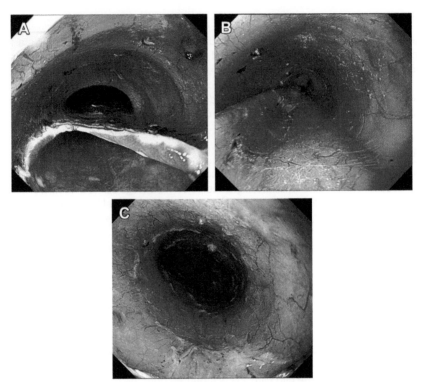

Fig. 7. (*A*) A submucosal tunnel is made from oral to anal, after mucosal incision. (*B*) The second tunnel is made at the opposite side, and the remaining submucosal fibers are dissected between the 2 tunnels. (*C*) Finally, en bloc ESD was completed.

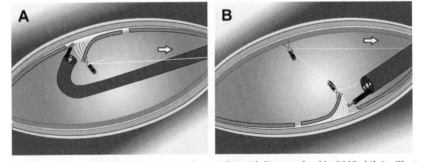

Fig. 8. The author and colleagues reported on a clip with line method in 2002. (*A*) An illustration showing clip with line method. A clip with line was placed at the edge of the target lesion when the circumferential incision was completed. Good counter traction and a clear field of vision were obtained when the line was pulled very gently. (*B*) The second clip can change the direction of traction. (*From* Oyama T, Yuichi K, Shimaya S, et al. Endoscopic mucosal resection using a hooking knife—intra gastric lesion lifting method. Stomach and Intestine 2002;37:1159. Japanese with English summary; with permission.)

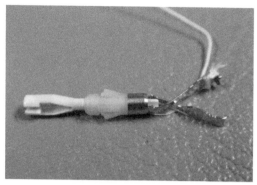

Fig. 9. A long, 3-0, silk line is tied to the arm part of the clip (HX-610-135, Olympus, Tokyo, Japan).

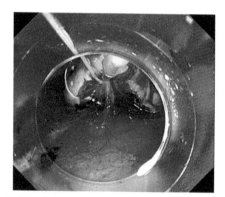

Fig. 10. The submucosal side of the target lesion is grasped by the clip.

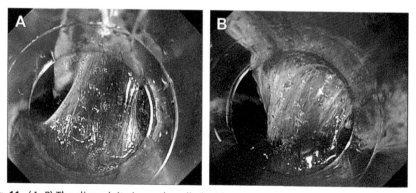

Fig. 11. (A, B) The clipped site is gently pulled with a traction line to provide countertraction to facilitate submucosal dissection.

HEMOSTASIS

Bleeding makes the visual field worse; therefore, hemostasis should be performed as soon as possible. When bleeding occurs during mucosal incision or dissection, the area should be flushed using a water jet system to find the origin of bleeding.

Hemostasis Using Knife

Hemostasis using an endoknife is useful for controlling oozing bleeds.[14,15] The tip of the knife is brought close to the origin, and electrical discharge is done with spray mode to obtain hemostasis (effect 2, 60 W).[15,16] Because prolonged electrical discharge may cause perforation, electrical discharge should be performed briefly. Therefore, it is important to maintain optimal distance using a transparent hood. A water jet system must be used to confirm the precise origin of the bleeding. A scope equipped with a water jet should be selected for esophageal ESD.

Hemostatic Procedures Using Hemostatic Forceps

Hemostatic forceps, such as FD-410LR (Olympus), are useful in cases of more active or spurting bleeding. After flushing with a water jet to locate the origin of the bleed, the origin is grasped with the hemostatic forceps. After that, reflushing with a water jet enables determination of whether the origin is grasped accurately. Then, the forceps are elevated a little to remove forceps from the proper muscular layer followed by electrical discharge with soft coagulation (effect 5, 40 W) to obtain hemostasis.

PREVENTION OF BLEEDING

Bleeding may worsen the visual field, leading to a higher risk of accidental complications. There are many vessels in the deep submucosal layer. A small vessel, 1 mm or less, could be cut using the Hook Knife without bleeding when spray coagulation mode is used (effect 2, 60 W). If the size of the vessel is 1 mm or larger, however, pre-cut coagulation should be performed to prevent bleeding (**Fig. 12A**). The large vessel is grasped by the hemostatic forceps (**Fig. 12B**) and is coagulated by soft coagulation (effect 5, 60 W). After that, the vessel can be cut using the Hook Knife and spray coagulation (effect 2, 60 W) without bleeding (**Fig. 12C**).

COMPLICATIONS

The major complication of EMR/ESD is perforation as well as air embolization and aspiration pneumonia. Perforations may cause mediastinal emphysema, which increases the mediastinal pressure crushing the esophageal lumen, leading to difficulty in securing the visual field. Severe mediastinal emphysema may be complicated by pneumothorax, which can lead to shock; therefore, electrocardiography, arterial oxygen saturation, and blood pressure (using an automated sphygmomanometer) monitoring should be conducted during ESD as well as periodic observation for subcutaneous emphysema through palpation. CO_2 insufflation is useful for preventing severe mediastinal emphysema.

Because the esophagus has no serous membrane and the intramediastinal pressure is lower than that of the esophageal lumen, mediastinal emphysema may appear without perforation. Dissection immediately above the proper muscular layer may damage the proper muscular layer during electrical discharge, which often causes mediastinal emphysema. Therefore, it is important to dissect the submucosal layer, making sure to leave the lowest one-third without exposure of the proper

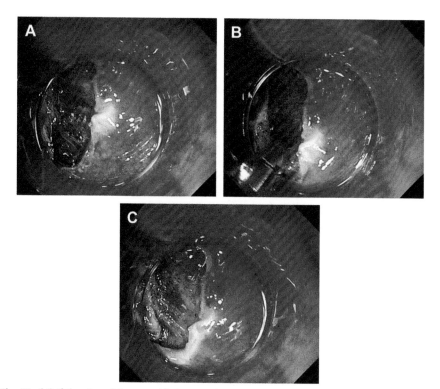

Fig. 12. (*A*) If the size of the vessel is 1 mm or lager, precut coagulation should be performed to prevent bleeding. (*B*) The large vessel is grasped by the hemostatic forceps and is coagulated by soft coagulation (effect 5, 60W). (*C*) After that, the vessel can be cut using the hook knife and spray coagulation (effect 2, 60) without bleeding.

muscular layer. Under intubation general anesthesia, the mediastinal pressure is higher than the intraesophageal pressure, enabling prevention of mediastinal emphysema and/or subcutaneous emphysema. Therefore, intubation general anesthesia is preferable for large lesions that are expected to take 2 or more hours for complete resection.

The perforation rate caused by esophageal EMR has been reported as 0% to 2.4 % and that of ESD as 0% to 6.4%.[7–10] The shape and size of perforation caused by EMR is different from that caused by ESD. Muscle removed by EMR can be 1 cm or larger, and sometimes closure by clips is difficult. On the other hand, the shape of perforation caused by ESD is linear, without defect of proper muscle. Therefore, closure by clips is usually easier than that of EMR. Sometimes, however, the clip may injure the remaining proper muscle and make the perforation larger. Therefore, operators should be skilled at clipping. Usually such perforations can be treated by fast insertion of a nasoesophageal tube and intravenous antibiotic administration, without surgery.

Water jets are useful for the detection of the bleeding point. Sometimes, however, water reflux causes aspiration pneumonia. A Flexible Overtube (Sumitomo Bakelite, Akita, Japan) is a useful device to prevent aspiration pneumonia. General anesthesia with tracheal intubation is necessary for the cervical esophageal ESD because the risk of aspiration pneumonia is high.

PREVENTION OF STRICTURE AFTER ESD

Stricture is a major complication after ESD. Multivariate analysis has shown that a mucosal defect of more than three-quarters of the circumference is a reliable predictor of stricture.[16–19] Post-ESD stricture substantially decreases patients' quality of life and requires multiple endoscopic balloon dilation (EBD) sessions. Preventive EBD has been the treatment of choice to prevent stricture; however, even after 6 sessions of preventive EBD, stricture is a frequent complication.

Recently, the efficacy of prophylactic oral prednisolone in the prevention of post-ESD stricture was described.[20] Although this method reduced the stricture rate, the cumulative dose of prednisolone was approximately 1000 mg, and exposure to such a high prednisolone dose raises concerns regarding adverse effects.

The efficacy of intralesional triamcinolone injection to prevent stricture after esophageal ESD has also been described.[21,22] Worth noting is research by Hanaoka and colleagues,[22] who studied the effect of a single session of intralesional steroid injections immediately after ESD. In this prospective study, they compared the results with a historical control group of patients who underwent ESD without intralesional steroid injection. The study group had a significantly lower stricture rate than historical control (10%, 3/30 patients in the study group, vs 66%, 19/29 patients in the control group; P<.0001) and a lower number of EBD sessions than historical control (median 0, range 0–2 vs median 2, range 0–15; P<.0001).

A unique method of preventing stricture after esophageal ESD has been published.[23] Specimens of oral mucosal tissue were collected from 9 patients with superficial esophageal neoplasms. Epithelial cell sheets were fabricated ex vivo by culturing isolated cells for 16 days on temperature-responsive cell culture surfaces. After a reduction in temperature, these sheets were endoscopically transplanted directly to the ulcer surfaces of patients who had just undergone ESD. Complete re-epithelialization occurred within a median time of 3.5 weeks. No patients experienced dysphagia, stricture, or other complications after the procedure, except for 1 patient who had a full circumferential ulceration that expanded to the esophagogastric junction.

SUMMARY

The advantage of ESD is the ability to achieve high R0 resection providing low local recurrence rate. Esophageal ESD is technically more difficult, however, than gastric ESD due to the narrower space of esophagus for endoscopic maneuvers. Also, the risk of perforation is higher because of the thin muscle layer of the esophageal wall. Blind dissection should be avoided to prevent perforation. A clip with line method is useful to keep good endoscopic view with countertraction. Only operators who have adequate skill should perform esophageal ESD.

REFERENCES

1. Makuuchi H. Endoscopic mucosal resection for early esophageal cancer: indication and techniques. Dig Endosc 1996;8:175–9.
2. Makuuchi H, Yoshida T, Ell C. Four-step endoscopic esophageal mucosal resection tube method of resection for early esophageal cancer. Endoscopy 2004;36:1013–8.
3. Inoue H, Takeshita K, Hori H, et al. Endoscopic mucosal resection with a cap-fitted panendoscope for esophagus, stomach and colon mucosal lesions. Gastrointest Endosc 1993;39:58–62.

4. Pech O, Gossner L, May A, et al. Endoscopic resection of superficial esophageal squamous-cell carcinomas: Western experience. Am J Gastroenterol 2004;99: 1226–32.

5. Momma K. Endoscopic treatment of esophageal mucosal carcinomas: indications and outcomes. Esophagus 2007;4:93–8.

6. Oyama T, Kikuchi Y. Aggressive endoscopic mucosal resection in the upper GI tract: hook knife EMR method. Minim Invasive Ther Allied Technol 2002; 11:291–5.

7. Oyama T, Tomori A, Hotta K, et al. Endoscopic submucosal dissection of early esophageal cancer. Clin Gastroenterol Hepatol 2005;3:S67–70.

8. Fujishiro M, Yahagi N, Kakushima N, et al. Endoscopic submucosal dissection of esophageal squamous cell neoplasms. Clin Gastroenterol Hepatol 2006;4: 688–94.

9. Ishihara R, Iishi H, Uedo N, et al. Comparison of EMR and endoscopic submucosal dissection for en bloc resection of early esophageal cancers in Japan. Gastrointest Endosc 2008;68:1066–72.

10. Takahashi H, Arimura Y, Hosokawa M, et al. Endoscopic submucosal dissection is superior to conventional endoscopic resection as a curative treatment for early squamous cell carcinoma, of the esophagus. Gastrointest Endosc 2010;71: 255–64.

11. Oyama T, Tomori A, Hotta K, et al. ESD with a hook knife for early esophageal cancer. Stomach Intestine 2006;41:491–7. Japanese with English summary.

12. Oyama T, Yuichi K, Shimaya S, et al. Endoscopic mucosal resection using a hooking knife – Intra gastric lesion lifting method. Stomach Intestine 2002;37:1155–61. Japanese with English summary.

13. Oyama T. Counter traction makes endoscopic submucosal dissection easier. Clin Endosc 2012;45:375–8.

14. Oyama T. Endoscopic submucosal dissection using a hook knife. Tech Gastrointest Endosc 2011;13:70–3.

15. Oyama T, Akihisa T, Hotta K, et al. Hemostasis with hook knife during Endoscopic submucosal dissection. Dig Endosc 2006;18:S128–30.

16. Katada C, Muto M, Manabe T, et al. Esophageal stenosis after endoscopic mucosal resection of superficial esophageal lesions. Gastrointest Endosc 2003; 57:165–9.

17. Mizuta H, Nishimori I, Kuratani Y, et al. Predictive factors for esophageal stenosis after endoscopic submucosal dissection for superficial esophageal cancer. Dis Esophagus 2009;22:626–31.

18. Ono S, Fujishiro M, Niimi K, et al. Predictors of postoperative stricture after esophageal endoscopic submucosal dissection for superficial esophageal squamous cell neoplasms. Endoscopy 2009;41:661–5.

19. Takahasi H, Arimura Y, Okahara S, et al. Risk of perforation during dilation for esophageal strictures after endoscopic resection in patients with early squamous cell carcinoma. Endoscopy 2011;43:184–9.

20. Yamaguchi N, Isomoto H, Nakayama T, et al. Usefulness of oral prednisolone in the treatment of esophageal stricture after endoscopic submucosal dissection for superficial esophageal squamous cell carcinoma. Gastrointest Endosc 2011;73:1115–21.

21. Hashimoto S, Kobayashi M, Takeuchi M, et al. The efficacy of endoscopic triamcinolone injection for the prevention of esophageal stricture after endoscopic submucosal dissection. Gastrointest Endosc 2011;74:1389–93.

22. Hanaoka N, Ishihara R, Takeuchi Y, et al. Intralesional steroid injection to prevent stricture after endoscopic submucosal dissection for esophageal cancer: a controlled prospective study. Endoscopy 2012;44:1007–11.

23. Ohki T, Yamato M, Ota M, et al. Prevention of esophageal stricture after endoscopic submucosal dissection using tissue-engineered cell sheets. Gastroenterology 2012;143:582–8.

Gastric ESD
Current Status and Future Directions of Devices and Training

Takuji Gotoda, MD, PhD, FASGE, FRCP[a],*, Khek-Yu Ho, MD, PhD[b],
Roy Soetikno, MD, MS, FASGE[c], Tonya Kaltenbach, MD, MS, FASGE[c],
Peter Draganov, MD, PhD, FASGE[d]

KEYWORDS

- Endoscopic submucosal dissection • Early gastric cancer • Lymph node metastasis
- Pathologic staging • Endoscopic mucosal resection

KEY POINTS

- ESD designed to provide precise pathologic staging and curability based on en bloc R0 specimen irrespective of the size and/or location of the tumor.
- ESD requires high technical skills on the part of the operator, is time consuming, and is associated with procedural related complications.
- Standardized ESD training system is urgently needed to disseminate safe and effective ESD technique to practices with limited ESD experience.

 Videos of endoscopic submucosal dissection procedures on the stomach accompany this article

PRINCIPLE OF ENDOSCOPIC RESECTION AS A DEFINITIVE TREATMENT

Early gastric cancer (EGC) is defined when the cancer invasion is confined to the mucosa or submucosa (T1 cancer), irrespective of the presence of lymph node

Disclosure Statement: Drs T. Gotoda, P. Draganov and K.-Y. Ho are lecturers for Olympus; Dr T. Gotoda is a lecturer for Pentax and Fujinon; Dr R. Soetikno is a lecturer and consultant for Olympus; Dr T. Kaltenbach is a grant recipient and consultant for Olympus.
[a] Department of Gastroenterology and Hepatology, Tokyo Medical University, 6-7-1, Nishishin-juku, Shinjuku-ku, Tokyo 160-0023, Japan; [b] Department of Medicine, Yong Loo Lin School of Medicine, National University of Singapore, Level 10, NUHS Tower Block, 1E Kent Ridge Road, Singapore 119228; [c] Department of Gastroenterology and Hepatology, Veterans Affairs Palo Alto, Stanford University, 3801 Miranda Avenue, GI-111, Palo Alto, CA 94304, USA; [d] Division of Gastroenterology, Hepatology and Nutrition, University of Florida, 1600 SW Archer Road, Room HD 602, PO Box 100214, Gainesville, FL 32610, USA
* Corresponding author.
E-mail address: takujigotoda@yahoo.co.jp

metastasis.[1] The presence of lymph node metastasis is a strong predictor on patients' prognosis,[2,3] and for this reason gastrectomy with lymph node dissection has historically been the gold standard for treatment of EGC.[4]

The 5-year cancer-specific survival rates of EGC limited to the mucosa or the superficial submucosa were reported to be 99% and 96%, respectively.[5] However, the traditional approach of radical gastric surgery is associated with significant morbidity and reductions in quality of life.[6] Surgery to remove intramucosal gastric cancer whereby the incidence of lymph node metastasis is low (up to 3%) is therefore excessive for most patients. By comparison, surgery in the majority is appropriate when the cancer involves the deep submucosa, where the incidence of lymph node metastasis increases to as high as 20%.[7] A stratification method to identify patients who have negligible risk for developing lymph node metastasis would thus optimize the selection of patients who can be cured by endoscopic resection and thus avoid the risks of surgery. The ideal patients for endoscopic resection rather than surgery are those who have a lower mortality risk from metastasis.[8]

Precise stratification of patients with favorable prognosis should be underscored. Endoscopic ultrasonography has limited staging accuracy (80%–90%),[9] and thus would result in unnecessary surgery in up to 20% of patients.[10–12] Ablation endoscopic techniques may cure EGC, but do not provide a pathologic specimen for analysis,[13] leaving the patient without proper staging or prognosis. Prior experience in the 1980s and 1990s suggests that pathologic staging is the best predictor of the risk for lymph node metastasis.[14,15]

The most accurate method to stratify the patients' prognosis for developing lymph node metastasis was reported by Gotoda and colleagues in 2000. In a study involving 5265 patients who had undergone gastrectomy with careful lymph node dissection and pathologic analysis, the risks of lymph node metastasis can be clustered to several pathologic findings of the involved mucosa and submucosa: macroscopic appearance, size, depth, differentiation of cancer, and lymphatic and vascular involvement. This seminal work provides one of the pillars of endoscopic resection of EGC.

The Paris classification of superficial neoplasias of the gastrointestinal tract provides another pillar. It allows standardization of the endoscopic appearance of EGC, which is then useful to estimate tumor depth and likelihood of the risk of lymph node metastasis.[16] The en bloc resected specimen provides further information on size, depth, and differentiation of cancer, as well as lymphatic and vascular involvement. Thus the tumor can be accurately staged, the patient's prognosis estimated, and the need for additional therapy assessed.[17,18]

The major advantage of endoscopic resection is the ability to provide accurate pathologic staging without precluding future surgical therapy.[19,20] After endoscopic resection, pathologic assessment of depth of cancer invasion, degree of cancer differentiation, and involvement of lymphatics or vessels allows the prediction of the risk of lymph node metastasis.[21] The endoscopic submucosal dissection (ESD) technique was developed to extend the ability of endoscopic mucosal resection (EMR) to remove lesions larger than 2 cm en bloc,[22,23] as EMR is limited to the resection of small tumors. It is also known that piecemeal resections of lesions larger than 2 cm lead to a high risk for recurrence of local cancer and inadequate pathologic staging.[24,25] ESD allows for large en bloc resection regardless of tumor size, location, and/or submucosal fibrosis, thereby allowing precise pathologic staging.[26–29] ESD is the most gratifying for patients with EGC because of its minimally invasive and curative potential, which is why it is increasingly used globally.[30–34]

INDICATIONS FOR ENDOSCOPIC RESECTION

The traditional criteria for endoscopic resection of EGC were founded on the technical limitation of EMR to remove gastric lesions of less than 2 cm in diameter en bloc.[35,36] The empirical indications for EMR include[37]: (1) papillary or tubular (differentiated) adenocarcinoma, (2) less than 2 cm in diameter, (3) without ulceration within tumor, and (4) no lymphatic-vascular involvement.

Clinical observations have noted, however, that the empirical indications for EMR were too strict and had led to unnecessary surgery. Therefore, expanded criteria for endoscopic resection have been proposed, especially after large en bloc resection became technically achievable using ESD.[38] The large number of patients included in the study reported by Gotoda and colleagues[39] was instrumental in defining the expanded criteria, as its 95% confidence intervals (CI) were narrow in comparison with the early studies with wide upper CI attributable to small sample sizes.[40–44] In addition, recent data showed that no lymph node metastasis was found in 310 patients with poorly differentiated adenocarcinoma and/or signet-ring cell EGC, less than 2 cm in diameter, without ulceration, and without lymphatics or vascular involvement (95% CI 0%–0.96%).[45] Therefore, patients with these finding may also be treated with ESD alone.

The longitudinal results of patients who were treated by endoscopic resections have provided the ultimate proof of its safety and efficacy. The long-term outcomes after EMR for small differentiated mucosal EGC less than 2 cm in diameter have been reported to be comparable with those following gastrectomy.[46–48] Patients who underwent ESD following the expanded criteria have long-term survival and outcomes similar to those of patients treated according to the traditional criteria.[49] The 5-year survival rate was 92% in patients in the traditional criteria group and 93% in the expanded criteria group. There was no significant difference in overall survival between these groups (multivariable hazard ratio 1.10; 95% CI 0.67–1.81).

The current indication of endoscopic resection for patients with EGC is called the Expanded Criteria for Endoscopic Resection in EGC (**Table 1**). The criteria are best used by comparing the risk for developing lymph node metastasis or distant metastasis against the risk of surgery, and considering patients' morbidities and preferences.[50,51] It is important to understand that the expanded criteria were developed to identify which patients have a low risk of lymph node metastasis. Patients meeting the criteria incur a risk of lymph node metastasis up to the upper limit of 95% CI.[52–54] This risk is by no means nonexistent (**Fig. 1**).

COMPLICATIONS

Although delayed bleeding is thought to be the most common complication, occurring in up to 8% of patients undergoing gastric ESD,[55] the risk of the procedure is primarily related to uncontrollable bleeding during ESD.[56] Acute bleeding may obscure the visual field, leading to a higher risk of complications. Therefore, endoscopic hemostasis should be immediately performed step by step (Videos 1 and 2). Small vessels can be coagulated using the ESD knife (forced coagulation mode, 50 W). Larger vessels should be coagulated by specially designed hemostatic forceps (FD-410LR; Olympus Medical Systems, Tokyo, Japan) using soft coagulation (80 W).[57]

After dissection has been completed, further hemostasis is performed on visible vessels to minimize delayed bleeding. The hemostatic forceps using soft coagulation are used to coagulate any visible small vessels.[58] Excessive coagulation in the area of the exposed muscle layer of the ESD defect should be avoided because of the risk of delayed perforation. Delayed bleeding, manifested by hematemesis or melena at 0 to 30 days after the procedure, is treated by emergent endoscopy, performed after

Table 1
Early gastric cancer with no risk of lymph node metastasis

Criteria	Incidence (No. with Metastasis/Total Number)	95% Confidence Interval
Intramucosal cancer	0/1230; 0%	0–0.3
Differentiated (well and/or moderately differentiated and/or papillary adenocarcinoma) type		
No lymphatic-vessel involvement		
Irrespective of ulcer findings		
Tumor size <3 cm		
Intramucosal cancer	0/929; 0%	0–0.4
Differentiated type		
No lymphatic-vessel involvement		
Without ulcer findings		
Irrespective of tumor size		
Intramucosal cancer	0/310; 0%	0–0.96
Undifferentiated (poorly differentiated adenocarcinoma and/or signet-ring cell carcinoma) type		
No lymphatic-vessel involvement		
Without ulcer findings		
Tumor size <2 cm		
Minute submucosal penetration (sm1)	0/145; 0%	0–2.5
Differentiated type		
No lymphatic-vessel involvement		
Tumor size <3 cm		

Data from Hirasawa T, Gotoda T, Miyata S, et al. Incidence of lymph node metastasis and the feasibility of endoscopic resection for undifferentiated-type early gastric cancer. Gastric Cancer 2009;12(3):148–52; and Uedo N, Iishi H, Tatsuta M, et al. Longterm outcomes after endoscopic mucosal resection for early gastric cancer. Gastric Cancer 2006;9(2):88–92.

resuscitation, using similar techniques (Video 3).[59] Delayed bleeding after ESD has been correlated with tumor location (lower part) and size.[60]

Perforations are typically closed by endoclips (Videos 4 and 5).[61,62] If pneumoperitoneum is significant, the patient may develop respiratory compromise or even shock (**Fig. 2**). Thus, to prevent the abdominal compartment syndrome, decompression of the pneumoperitoneum must be immediately performed using a 14-gauge puncture needle with side slits after confirmation, using a 23-gauge needle syringe filled with saline (Video 6). Nasogastric suction is applied for 12 hours and broad-spectrum antibiotic is given for 2 days. Bacterial peritonitis is relatively rare because of the antibacterial effect of gastric acid. Diet is slowly advanced on day 3 or day 4 after ESD.

To prevent gastric perforations and better facilitate ESD, polyethylene glycol or sodium hyaluronate as an injection agent has recently been reported. These agents remain longer in the submucosa and create clearer dissection layer.[63–65] No evidence of peritoneal dissemination and/or lymph node metastasis caused by gastric perforation has been reported.[66] The use of CO_2 to insufflate the stomach during ESD is also extremely useful, as CO_2 is readily absorbed should perforation occur.

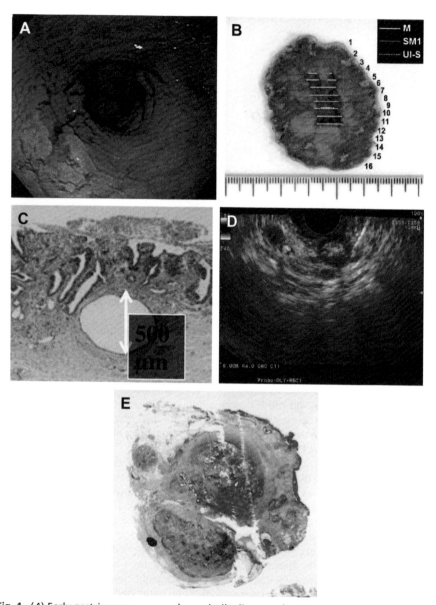

Fig. 1. (*A*) Early gastric cancer was endoscopically diagnosed as IIc T1a. (*B*) En bloc resection by endoscopic submucosal dissection (ESD). (*C*) IIc T1b (500 μm submucosal penetration) with negative horizontal and vertical margins classified into the expanded indication. (*D*) Regional lymph node metastasis was confirmed by endoscopic ultrasound-guided fine-needle aspiration 32 months after ESD. (*E*) Curative radical surgery with only 1 lymph node metastasis was achieved.

DIAGNOSIS

Accurate diagnosis of the lateral and vertical margins of EGC is important before endoscopic resection. Similarly to the colon, for which patient preparation is critical, a clean upper gastrointestinal tract is also hugely important. Mucus and debris need

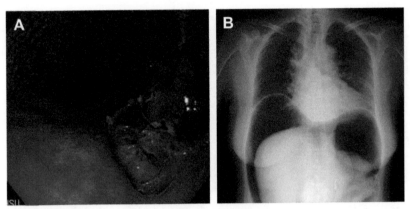

Fig. 2. (A) Perforation on the greater curve of antrum during submucosal dissection by insulated-tip (IT) knife. (B) Pneumoperitoneum causing possible abdominal component syndrome.

to be removed before and during the examination. In Japan, mucolytic and defoaming agents are used. In Western countries, acetylcysteine may be used as a mucolytic and activated dimethicone as a defoaming agent.

Most EGC are nonpolypoid, and the depressed type is the most common. Several endoscopic findings suggest submucosal invasion in a depressed EGC: thickening, rigidity, disappearance of mucosal surface pattern, extensive redness, or nodularity within the depression, and swelling of converging folds. Whereas the larger depressed EGC are more likely to be submucosal, size is not predictive of submucosal invasion in the flat ones. Moreover, the prediction of submucosal involvement in the ulcerated type is more difficult because of the presence of fibrosis, which may mimic some of the findings described in the depressed lesions. Endoscopic ultrasonography is rarely used to estimate the depth of the lesion.

Indigo carmine chromoendoscopy is the most useful method to determine the lateral margin of EGC. The appearance of the lesion is readily seen and relatively easily understood. Its use allows the determination of the macroscopic appearance and size of the lesion. At the time of diagnosis, the lesion is biopsied at its worst-appearing portion to confirm and document the diagnosis. Multiple biopsies of the lesion are avoided because of the risk of inducing undue submucosal fibrosis, which would make endoscopic resection difficult. Normal surrounding mucosa is biopsied separately to confirm that the assessment of the lateral margin is correct. Lesions that meet the expanded criteria are candidates for endoscopic resection.

Narrow-band imaging (NBI) has increasingly been described as an alternative to indigo carmine image enhancement, especially for the diagnosis of small, depressed, or flat types of EGC. However, its application requires high magnification, which is not available worldwide. In addition, NBI is not applicable for determining the lateral extent of undifferentiated types of EGC. The vessel plus surface classification system, which has been well studied by Yao and colleagues,[67] is based on the ability to visualize both the microvascular and microsurface patterns.

TRAINING

The learning and application of these relatively complex endoscopic therapeutic techniques for early gastric cancer have been demonstrated across the world. Most

Japanese experts set the level of expertise at 50 to 100 cases to become proficient in gastric ESD,[68] and require a trainee to perform at least 30 gastric ESD cases under the supervision of an expert to gain basic proficiency in this technique.[69,70] Fundamental skills and knowledge of the macroscopic diagnosis, indications, tools, and techniques, as well as the resection specimen for histologic preparation and interpretation, should be sought through self-education seminars and conferences. Participation in hands-on courses with isolated or live animal stomach and live demonstrations is vital in accelerating the learning curve. In comparison with the self-taught method, specialty centers that use a standard of practice to systematically provide training and competency under direct expert supervision have been more successful.

A standardized ESD training system is urgently needed to disseminate a safe and effective ESD technique to practices with limited ESD experience. A questionnaire survey of Japanese experts reported that ESD training should be conducted in a step-up approach after prior experience with conventional EMR. The panel concluded that preceptees should observe and attend ESD procedures as an assistant in at least 20 and 5 cases, respectively, so as to understand a wide variety of ESD procedures and strategies and to develop trouble-shooting abilities.[71] The trainee should start with an antral lesion of less than 20 mm in diameter without ulcer, as it has the lowest risk of noncurative resection, and then progress to lesions in the distal and proximal stomach.[72] Submucosal dissection has been shown to be more difficult than mucosal incision, mostly because of uncontrollable hemorrhage.[56] As such, appropriate supervision by a highly experienced endoscopist is necessary in the early phase of learning, because a significant number of cases require the supervisor to complete the procedure after uncontrollable hemorrhage or perforation occurs. Choi and colleagues[48] highlighted the difficulties in learning such novel complex techniques independently without the direction of an experienced mentor. These investigators reported an initial complete resection rate of 60% to 65% and an en bloc resection rate of 45% to 55% with 3 perforations. Of note, neither years of prior endoscopic experience, number of endoscopic procedures per year, nor prior experience with endoscopic retrograde cholangiopancreatography has been associated with a significant difference in the risk of perforation during training.[73]

Western ESD experts to supervise ESD training are limited in number, and virtual simulators for ESD are not yet available. Thus the use of animal models to facilitate the early training of ESD is important to minimize the risk of higher complications at the beginning of the learning curve in humans. Proper use of ex vivo and in vivo animal models is performed in an animal facility under the direction of a veterinarian, with dedicated equipment and a standardized setup.[74] Parra-Blanco and colleagues[75] demonstrated an effective learning strategy of the Western endoscopist by training in ESD in the absence of expert supervision. Indeed, Parra-Blanco learned ESD from Japanese experts, but then trained in harvested pig stomachs and then in live pigs, and reported a 4.5% (95% CI 0.12%–22.8%) perforation rate.[75] A European group[76] assessed the impact on 18 experienced endoscopists (39% with basic ESD experience) who participated in a 2-day training course that included seminars and hands-on training with living pigs, and was supervised by experts in ESD. Each endoscopist performed a mean 4.1 ESD, mostly in the stomach (84%), with a perforation rate of 22%. Although technical maneuvers may be simulated using a pig model, anatomic differences between the pig and human stomach may pose limitations to training. Although compared with humans the pig model in gastric ESD exhibits less frequent bleeding, more difficult submucosal injection, and less fibrosis,[75] the use of models allows endoscopists to ascend the learning curve in a relatively short time, and enhance the safety and efficacy of the patient experience.

PRACTICAL APPROACH

The low prevalence of superficial gastric epithelial neoplasms has translated into very few opportunities for Western endoscopists to perform gastric ESD.[77–81] The first dedicated ESD devices were approved in the United States less than 2 years ago. Furthermore, the choice of devices, endoscopes, and ancillary equipment for ESD available in the United States is different to that available in Japan. Finally, the technical expertise, training opportunities, and backgrounds of endoscopists embarking on ESD in the West differ significantly from those of their Eastern counterparts.[69] This section reviews the technical aspects of gastric ESD from a Western perspective.

Endoscopes and Endoscope Accessories

Standard upper endoscopes with water-jet function are adequate for most cases. Water-jet irrigation is highly advantageous because it can facilitate identification of bleeding vessels. Some experts recommend the use of specialized endoscopes because of perceived advantages (therapeutic channel endoscope for better suction, double-channel endoscope to pass 2 devices simultaneously to save time on device exchanges, double-bending endoscope to facilitate access to some difficult-to-reach lesions). The authors favor the use of standard-size endoscopes because of their small diameter and ease of maneuverability.

A specialized soft, clear plastic distal attachment (cap) should be applied to all endoscopes for ESD. For each endoscope model there is a corresponding size of cap (JMDN 38819001; TOP Corp, Tokyo, Japan). The use of CO_2 for insufflation is highly recommended because it causes less luminal distention and patient discomfort. Furthermore, if there is a perforation the leaking CO_2 will rapidly be reabsorbed from the peritoneal cavity, thus decreasing the risk of respiratory compromise caused by increased intraperitoneal pressure. With the use of CO_2, the ESD can be completed after the perforation has been closed using endoscopic clips.[82]

Dedicated ESD Devices

A large number of devices for ESD are now available in Japan[83,84] and are divided into 2 general categories: needle-knife type and scissors type. The needle-knife devices can be further subdivided into uncovered type and insulated type. Only a limited number of needle-type devices are approved by the Food and Drug Administration, and at present none of the scissors types is available in the United States.

There are 6 basic functions required from a device at the time of ESD: mucosal marking, submucosal injection, precutting (the very first small incision into the mucosa needed to engage all insulated-tip [IT] type devices), cutting of the circumferential incision, submucosal dissection, and hemostasis. The ESD devices available in the United States and the type of function that they can accomplish are summarized in **Table 2**. It should be emphasized that although a knife can be used to perform a specific function extremely well, it does not necessarily make the device functionally suitable in all circumstances.

The IT2 (KD-611L; Olympus America Inc, Center Valley, PA, USA) is an IT knife which, at present, is the only insulated device available for gastric ESD in the United States. The Dual knife (KD-650L; Olympus America Inc) is a needle-knife device that has 2 positions: retracted and extended. An important property is that the needle protrudes 0.3 mm beyond the protective catheter even when the knife is in the retracted position, and 2 mm when extended. This function allows the knife to be used for marking and hemostasis (retracted) and for precutting, circumferential incision, and submucosal dissection (extended). The Hook knife (upper length

Table 2
ESD devices and their functions

Device	Marking	Injection	Precutting	Circumferential Incision	Submucosal Dissection	Hemostasis
IT2				✔	✔	✔
Dual	✔		✔	✔	✔	✔
Hook	✔		✔	✔	✔	✔
Hybrid	✔	✔	✔	✔	✔	✔
Coagulating forceps						✔

KD-620LR; Olympus America Inc) has an L-shaped tip, which is useful to hook tissue and subsequently cut it. The Hook knife is usually used to dissect fibrotic tissue under some EGC procedures. The Hybrid knife (ERBE USA, Marietta, GA, USA) allows submucosal injection and also cutting, therefore making it suitable for all stages of ESD, with potential time savings resulting from fewer device exchanges. The ultrafine water jet issuing from the tip of the knife will penetrate the mucosa but cannot penetrate the proper muscle layer. Therefore the fluid accumulates in the submucosa, creating a submucosal cushion. A dedicated computerized unit (ERBE Jet) is required to operate the jet function, which adds to the cost of capital equipment required for ESD.

Coagulating hot forceps are also required. All described knives can provide hemostasis for smaller vessels, but for larger bleeding vessels, dedicated monopolar coagulating forceps are usually needed. Dedicated hemostatic forceps (Coag grasper, FD-410LR; Olympus America Inc) are available, although in the stomach, the authors favor the use of standard hot biopsy forceps (Boston Scientific Corp, Natick, MA, USA) because their larger size of cup with serrated jaws can be used to provide better hemostasis.

Injection Agents

Sodium hyaluronate solution is typically used in Japan, but very high cost has restricted its application in the United States.[85] Normal saline can be used for smaller lesions, but frequent repeat injections may be needed. The authors favor the use of a mixture containing 85 mL of normal saline with hydroxypropyl methylcellulose and indigo carmine (Gonak 2.5%; Akorn Inc, Somerset, NJ, USA), which has been proved safe when used for EMR.[86] Methylene blue should not be used, owing to its potential for complications and because it is absorbed into the cell nucleus, which results in intense staining that hampers visualization.[87]

Electrosurgical Generator and Generator Settings

A computerized electrosurgical generator providing modulated current options is essential for a successful ESD procedure. The generators available in the United States that are suitable for ESD are the ICC 200E, VIO 200S, and VIO 300D (ERBE USA), and the ESG 100 (Olympus America Inc). The recommended settings (type of modulated current, power output, effect, duration, and so forth) are different for different stages of the procedure, type of instrument used, location of the lesion, and different models of generators. In addition, multiple other variables can significantly contribute to the final tissue effect, including the surface area of the device electrode in contact with the tissue, the speed of movement of the electrode, the pressure applied with the electrode, the presence of coagulated tissue debris sticking to the electrode, the target tissue itself (fibrotic vs high water content), and grounding-pad placement (the pad should be placed on the patient's flank rather than the lower extremity). As a result, the recommended generator settings vary greatly among experts performing ESD. Therefore, although settings recommended by experts will be a good starting point, the final tissue effect will greatly depend on a multitude of factors, most importantly the individual endoscopist's ESD technique.

ESD Planning Strategy

The initial important step is to determine the most appropriate therapeutic modality for a specific lesion and specific patient. In the United States, a multidisciplinary approach (eg, consensus from multidisciplinary tumor board) is strongly encouraged. If ESD is to be carried out, a well-planned strategy is essential for procedural success. This strategy should include plans for sedation, management of antiplatelet drugs or anticoagulants, need for additional consultations (eg, cardiology in patients with defibrillators and so forth), need for special equipment, and need for preprocedure and/or postprocedure hospital admissions. A lesion-specific strategy should also be outlined ahead of time, which should include selection of ESD device, type of submucosal injection fluid, site of initial precut incision, order and degree of the circumferential incision (complete vs partial), and direction of the submucosal dissection, among other factors.

Procedural Steps

Determining the lateral extent of the lesion
The use of indigo carmine chromoendoscopy and, in select cases, NBI, is essential at this stage (Video 7).

Mucosal markings
Mucosal markings are placed 5 mm lateral to the lesion margin using a device suitable for this function (**Fig. 3**A). In addition, the use of argon plasma coagulation for marking is convenient, but will add to the cost of the procedure.

Submucosal injection
Typically the injection is done in stages; only injecting the area that needs to be incised. Unlike during EMR, the goal is not to initially lift the lesion itself, but to lift the perimeter of the lesion to allow the circumferential incision. Adequate injection is needed, but a very large volume of injection is to be avoided because it may compromise access to the lesion.

Initial mucosal incision (precutting)
If an IT2 knife is to be used for the circumferential incision (the authors' preferred approach), a small initial mucosal incision (precutting) is first made to gain access to the submucosal space. The authors favor the use of the Dual knife for this step. The precutting incision should be deep enough to allow access to the submucosal space, but at the same time not too deep to injure the muscularis propria (see **Fig. 3**B). The exact location of the initial mucosal incision is determined by multiple factors (oral vs anal side, access to the lesion in forward vs retroflex view, dependent vs nondependent site, the type of device that will be used in the later stages of ESD). Because circumferential incision with the IT2 can be easier to accomplish when moving the knife toward the scope than moving the knife laterally, more than 1 precut incision may be needed.

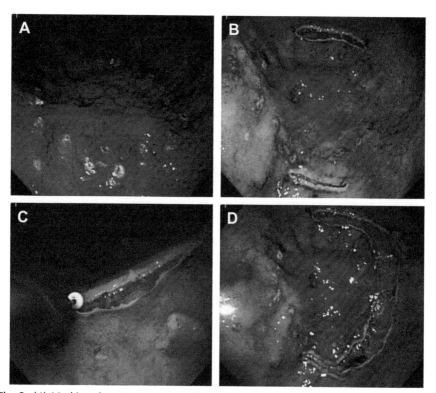

Fig. 3. (*A*) Marking dots 5 mm around the tumor margin. (*B*) Lateral incisions using Dual knife at 12 o'clock and 6 o'clock after enough submucosal cushion. (*C*) Mucosal incision 5 mm lateral to the mucosal markings by IT2 knife. (*D*) Halfway into mucosal incision. (*E*) Complete circumferential mucosal incision. (*F*) Reinjection of fluid should be carried out to maintain adequate submucosal cushion. (*G*) Reinjection just above the proper muscle layer because of the loosest connecting tissue. (*H*) Cap facilitates opening of submucosal layer. (*I*) Parallel movement of IT2 knife for muscle layer. (*J*) Gravity should be always considered.

Circumferential incision

The circumferential incision is carried out 5 mm lateral to the mucosal markings to give a total of 10 mm normal tissue margin (5 mm from the lateral margin of the lesion to the marking and 5 additional millimeters for the circumferential incision) (see **Fig. 3**C–E). The sequence and direction of the incision is determined by the lesion location and selection of the devices (eg, a pulling motion is used with the IT knife, whereas a pushing motion is typically used with the noninsulated type of needle knives). In some cases it may be advantageous not to carry out a full initial circumferential incision to facilitate access to the lesion.

Submucosal dissection

The exact technique of submucosal dissection varies among endoscopists and differs significantly for the different devices and degree of submucosal fibrosis, but few general considerations apply. The correct plane for dissection should be recognized before every cut. Fluid should be reinjected to maintain adequate submucosal cushion (see **Fig. 3**F). The preferred site for reinjection is just above the proper muscle layer (see **Fig. 3**G, H). The position of the accessory channel should be factored in when

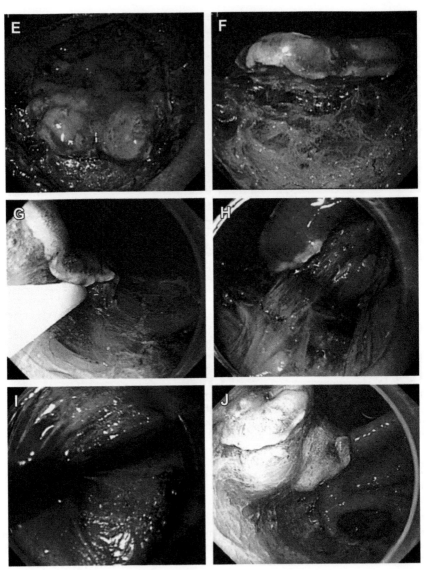

Fig. 3. (continued)

approaching the lesion. The site where the device will exit the scope should be positioned at the target, rather than first bringing the device out and then repositioning the tip to the area of interest. For submucosal dissection, the parallel movement for muscle layer with the IT2 is typically lateral (eg, slicing motion as seen with a Japanese samurai sword) (see **Fig. 3I**) and with the Dual knife forward (eg, stabbing motion as seen with a Western-style straight sword or dagger). In any event, it is essential to maintain a submucosal dissection plane through the submucosal layer while avoiding injury to the proper muscle layer or the specimen. Adequate reinjection of fluid into the submucosa, using the distal attachment as a retractor, use of suction/insufflation, and use of gravity all can greatly facilitate this task. The direction of gravity should be factored in when planning the specific ESD strategy for a particular lesion (see **Fig. 3J**).

INNOVATIONS FOR ESD
Limitations of Current Standard Endoscopic Surgical Systems

Although ESD is a well-accepted minimally invasive procedure for removal of early-stage malignant gastrointestinal lesions, the procedure requires high technical skills on the part of the endoscopist, is time consuming, and is associated with a high rate of procedurally related complications. The major problem lies in the lack of a suitable endoscopic platform and instruments for its performance. Conventional endoscopes were initially never designed to support the performance of intricate procedures such as ESD. Operation of current endoscopy systems suffers from a severe lack of dexterity. Precision in maneuvers is very difficult to achieve, resulting sometimes in inadvertent incisions leading to bleeding, and even perforation of the gastrointestinal wall. As all current standard endoscopic instruments are deployed on a single axis in line with the endoscope, off-axis motions such as the triangulation of surgical instruments are rendered almost impossible.

In addition, owing to the sheer length of the endoscope, and the often-winding gastrointestinal tract it has to negotiate, the force transmission from the operator is diminished by the time it reaches the target, resulting in insufficient force for effectual traction, countertraction, and dissection of the tissue. In ensuring a safe submucosal dissection of a target lesion, it is extremely important that the operator steers the knife parallel to and above the muscularis propria. This maneuver is particularly challenging with the visibility of the dissecting plane not always being ideal, as the illumination source of today's standard endoscope is fixed at the distal tip of the endoscope. As the light source moves with the endoscope, it is almost impossible for the endoscopist to focus the light on the surgical field. Furthermore, with CO_2 insufflations manually controlled through the endoscope, continuous maintenance of optimal internal pressure to maintain luminal space and full view of the surgical field is not easy. Thus, ESD remains a procedure restricted only to those who are highly skilled in performing intricate endoscopic interventions.

Recent Innovations in ESD Instrumentations and Future Possibilities

In recent years, several innovations providing solutions for easier and safer performance of ESD have emerged, with a few having been commercialized since. Most of these innovations are in the form of auxiliary devices designed to overcome specific technical limitations of current ESD instrumentation, although a few are completely modified therapeutic systems enhanced and/or redesigned to support the performance not only of endoscopic procedures.

Auxiliary endoscopic devices developed thus far address only specific technical shortcomings of currently used therapeutic endoscopic systems. Most notably, the Japanese endoscope manufacturer, Olympus, has introduced the Endolifter, a dedicated retraction device designed specifically to support the performance of ESD.[88] The Endolifter makes possible simultaneous grasping, retracting, and lifting of the mucosa during ESD, resulting in better visualization of the cutting line in the submucosal tissue layer. Other innovations providing similar benefits include the most recent Endo-Dissector, a German prototype instrument designed specifically for ESD,[89] and the Maryland dissector manufactured in the United States.[90] Other devices designed to facilitate adequate exposure of the submucosal layer during ESD include a grasping-type scissors forceps (GSF) to grasp and lift the submucosa,[91] a rubber strip–based traction device (S-O clip), which when applied to the colon wall enables traction on the edge of the lesion,[92] an Impact Shooter (TOP Corp, Japan), which when deployed with the usual therapeutic endoscope provides a 2-point fixed ESD system that allows expansion of the mucosal dissection surface to ensure a sufficient visual field throughout the ESD procedure,[93] and an externally deployed magnetic controlling device to facilitate magnetic anchor-guided ESD (MAG-ESD) through mucosal lifting for gastric submucosal dissection.[94]

Several other innovations have focused on redesigning the endoscope to provide a more versatile endoscopic platform to support the performance of ESD as well as other complex surgical procedures such as NOTES (Natural Orifice Transluminal Endoscopic Surgery). The most basic among these are modified endoscopic systems such as the double-channel therapeutic endoscope, called the R-Scope (Olympus Japan).[95] The double-channel therapeutic R-scope is built with 2 movable deflecting instrument channels to facilitate better access and orientation of surgical tools. More advanced systems include multitasking endoscopic platforms such as the EndoSA-MURAI (Olympus Japan),[96] the Direct Drive Endoscopic system (DDES) (Boston Scientific),[97] and the TransPort Multi-lumen Operating Platform (USGI Medical, San Clemente, CA, USA).[98]

The EndoSAMURAI is designed with 2 additional independent flexible channels besides the usual working channel to allow convenient independent deployment of interchangeable surgical instruments. Similarly, the DDES is equipped with 3 working channels for multifunction instrumentation, together with an ergonomically designed user interface, while the Anubis (advanced flexible natural orifice translu-minal endoscopic surgery platform) permits the deployment of 3 end-effectors with multifunctional advanced capabilities, and allows triangulation of equipment along the optical field. These devices increase the control of surgical effectors manipulating the target tissue, and enhance performance in complex surgical tasks.

Although all the aforementioned innovations are significant improvements over the current endoscopy systems, these new platforms still fall short of providing a complete solution to the technical problems faced by therapeutic endoscopists today. The solution in sight probably lies in robotics. In the first attempt of its kind, Phee and colleagues[99,100] designed a novel robotic-enhanced Master And Slave Translumi-nal Endoscopic Robot (MASTER) (**Fig. 4**A). Unlike the other contemporary innovations, MASTER uses robotic technology to facilitate full instrumental mobility, and completely separates the control of end-effector motion from that of endoscopic movement. Surgical tasks are instead independently and intuitively executed by a second operator via a human-machine interface. This interface enables bimanual coordination of interchangeable effector instruments to facilitate actions such as retraction/exposure, traction/countertraction, and approximation and dissection of tissue. As robotics allow the slave effectors to be deployed off-axis from the endo-scope, triangulation of surgical end-effectors, a step essential for any surgery, is made easy. Through the master-slave system, significant force could be exerted to the point of action, allowing the end-effectors to effectively manipulate and dissect the tissue. Furthermore, with the enhancement of haptic feedback, the operator can obtain a sense of touch and force at the effector end to help in the appropriate control of application of force at the surgical target.

Thus far, trials conducted in animals and human subjects have shown that MASTER is a promising platform for efficient performance of complex endoluminal surgery such as ESD.[100,101] In its first clinical trial in humans, 5 patients with EGC successfully underwent ESD using MASTER. All lesions were successfully resected en bloc, with a mean submucosal dissection time of 18.6 minutes (median, 16 minutes; range, 3–50 minutes) (see **Fig. 4**B).[102] Three patients were discharged from the hospital

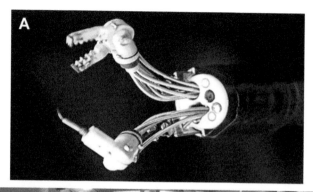

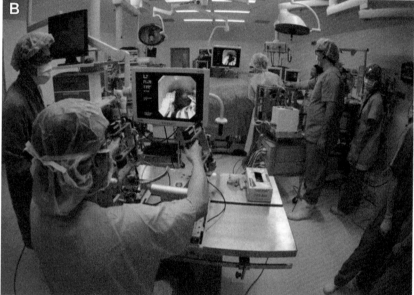

Fig. 4. (*A*) MASTER system. (*B*) Surgeon and endoscopist using the prototype robot in a human trial.

within 12 hours and the other 2 patients were discharged 3 days after the procedure. No complication was found at the 30-day follow-up examination.

MASTER is currently being further developed with an array of auxiliary devices and swappable end-effectors to support both endoluminal and transluminal endoscopic surgery. A dedicated suturing system for safe luminal closure with MASTER is in early development. In terms of providing a safe surgical environment within the abdomen, the use of MASTER with steady-pressure automatically controlled endoscopy (SPACE),[103] a novel platform for flexible gastrointestinal endoscopy developed by ENGINE (Endeavor for Next Generation of INterventional Endoscopy) in Japan, is currently being explored. It is envisaged that when ready, MASTER together with SPACE (MASTER-SPACE), and a complete armamentarium of new adaptable devices and swappable end-effectors, will adequately enable the efficient and safe performance of endoluminal procedures such as ESD.

SUPPLEMENTARY DATA

Videos related to this article can be found online at http://dx.doi.org/10.1016/j.giec. 2013.11.009.

REFERENCES

1. Japanese Gastric Cancer Association. Japanese classification of gastric carcinoma: 3rd English edition. Gastric Cancer 2011;14:101–12.
2. Itoh H, Oohata Y, Nakamura K, et al. Complete ten-year postgastrectomy followup of early gastric cancer. Am J Surg 1989;158:14–6.
3. Ohta H, Noguchi Y, Takagi K, et al. Early gastric carcinoma with special reference to macroscopic classification. Cancer 1987;60:1099–106.
4. Sano T, Sasako M, Kinoshita T, et al. Recurrence of early gastric cancer. Followup of 1475 patients and review of the Japanese literature. Cancer 1993;72: 3174–8.
5. Sasako M, Kinoshita T, Maruyama K. Prognosis of early gastric cancer. Stomach and Intestine 1993;23:139–46.
6. Sasako M. Risk factors for surgical treatment in the Dutch Gastric Cancer Trial. Br J Surg 1997;84:1567–71.
7. Sano T, Kobori O, Muto T. Lymph node metastasis from early gastric cancer: endoscopic resection of tumour. Br J Surg 1992;79:241–4.
8. Ludwig K, Klautke G, Bernhard J, et al. Minimally invasive and local treatment for mucosal early gastric cancer. Surg Endosc 2005;19:1362–6.
9. Sano T, Okuyama Y, Kobori O, et al. Early gastric cancer. Endoscopic diagnosis of depth of invasion. Dig Dis Sci 1990;35:1340–4.
10. Saitoh Y, Obara T, Watari J, et al. Invasion depth diagnosis of depressed type early colorectal cancers by combined use of videoendoscopy and chromoendoscopy. Gastrointest Endosc 1998;48:362–70.
11. Ohashi S, Segawa K, Okamura S, et al. The utility of endoscopic ultrasonography and endoscopy in the endoscopic mucosal resection of early gastric cancer. Gut 1999;45:599–604.
12. Akahoshi K, Chijiwa Y, Hamada S, et al. Pretreatment staging of endoscopically early gastric cancer with a 15 MHz ultrasound catheter probe. Gastrointest Endosc 1998;48:470–6.
13. Kitamura T, Tanabe S, Koizumi W, et al. Argon plasma coagulation for early gastric cancer: technique and outcome. Gastrointest Endosc 2006;63:48–54.
14. Hull MJ, Mino-Kenudson M, Nishioka NS, et al. Endoscopic mucosal resection: an improved diagnostic procedure for early gastroesophageal epithelial neoplasms. Am J Surg Pathol 2006;30:114–8.
15. Ahmad NA, Kochman ML, Long WB, et al. Efficacy, safety, and clinical outcomes of endoscopic mucosal resection: a study of 101 cases. Gastrointest Endosc 2002;55:390–6.
16. The Paris endoscopic classification of superficial neoplastic lesions: esophagus, stomach, and colon: November 30 to December 1. Gastrointest Endosc 2002;58:S3–43.
17. Nagano H, Ohyama S, Fukunaga T, et al. Indications for gastrectomy after incomplete EMR for early gastric cancer. Gastric Cancer 2005;8:149–54.
18. Yano H, Kimura Y, Iwazawa T, et al. Laparoscopic management for local recurrence of early gastric cancer after endoscopic mucosal resection. Surg Endosc 2005;19:981–5.

19. Yanai H, Matsubara Y, Kawano T, et al. Clinical impact of strip biopsy for early gastric cancer. Gastrointest Endosc 2004;60:771–7.
20. Farrell JJ, Lauwers GY, Okamoto T, et al. Endoscopic mucosal resection using a cap-fitted endoscope improves tissue resection and pathology interpretation: an animal study. Gastric Cancer 2006;9:3–8.
21. Gotoda T, Sasako M, Ono H, et al. Evaluation of the necessity for gastrectomy with lymph node dissection for patients with submucosal invasive gastric cancer. Br J Surg 2001;88:444–9.
22. Korenaga D, Haraguchi M, Tsujitani S, et al. Clinicopathological features of mucosal carcinoma of the stomach with lymph node metastasis in eleven patients. Br J Surg 1986;73:431–3.
23. Ell C, May A, Gossner L, et al. Endoscopic mucosal resection of early cancer and high-grade dysplasia in Barrett's esophagus. Gastroenterology 2000;118:670–7.
24. Tanabe S, Koizumi W, Mitomi H, et al. Clinical outcome of endoscopic aspiration mucosectomy for early stage gastric cancer. Gastrointest Endosc 2002;56: 708–13.
25. Kim JJ, Lee JH, Jung HY, et al. EMR for early gastric cancer in Korea: a multicenter retrospective study. Gastrointest Endosc 2007;66:693–700.
26. Hirao M, Masuda K, Asanuma T, et al. Endoscopic resection of early gastric cancer and other tumors with local injection of hypertonic saline-epinephrine. Gastrointest Endosc 1988;34:264–9.
27. Ono H, Kondo H, Gotoda T, et al. Endoscopic mucosal resection for treatment of early gastric cancer. Gut 2001;48:225–9.
28. Hosokawa K, Yoshida S. Recent advances in endoscopic mucosal resection for early gastric cancer. Gan To Kagaku Ryoho 1998;25:476–83 [in Japanese].
29. Yokoi C, Gotoda T, Hamanaka H, et al. Endoscopic submucosal dissection allows curative resection of locally recurrent early gastric cancer after prior endoscopic mucosal resection. Gastrointest Endosc 2006;64:212–8.
30. Rembacken BJ, Gotoda T, Fujii T, et al. Endoscopic mucosal resection. Endoscopy 2001;33:709–18.
31. Soetikno RM, Gotoda T, Nakanishi Y, et al. Endoscopic mucosal resection. Gastrointest Endosc 2003;57:567–79.
32. Gotoda T. Endoscopic resection of early gastric cancer. Gastric Cancer 2007; 10:1–11.
33. Gotoda T, Yamamoto H, Soetikno RM. Endoscopic submucosal dissection of early gastric cancer. J Gastroenterol 2006;41:929–42.
34. Jung HY. Endoscopic resection for early gastric cancer: current status in Korea. Dig Endosc 2012;24(Suppl 1):159–65.
35. Yamao T, Shirao K, Ono H, et al. Risk factors for lymph node metastasis from intramucosal gastric carcinoma. Cancer 1996;77:602–6.
36. Tsujitani S, Oka S, Saito H, et al. Less invasive surgery for early gastric cancer based on the low probability of lymph node metastasis. Surgery 1999;125:148–54.
37. Japanese gastric cancer treatment guidelines 2010 (ver. 3). Gastric Cancer 2011;14:113–23.
38. Soetikno R, Kaltenbach T, Yeh R, et al. Endoscopic mucosal resection for early cancers of the upper gastrointestinal tract. J Clin Oncol 2005;23:4490–8.
39. Gotoda T, Yanagisawa A, Sasako M, et al. Incidence of lymph node metastasis from early gastric cancer: estimation with a large number of cases at two large centers. Gastric Cancer 2000;3:219–25.
40. Hiki Y. Endoscopic mucosal resection (EMR) for early gastric cancer. Nihon Geka Gakkai Zasshi 1996;97:273–8 [in Japanese].

41. Ohgami M, Otani Y, Kumai K, et al. Laparoscopic surgery for early gastric cancer. Nihon Geka Gakkai Zasshi 1996;97:279–85 [in Japanese].

42. Yasuda K, Shiraishi N, Suematsu T, et al. Rate of detection of lymph node metastasis is correlated with the depth of submucosal invasion in early stage gastric carcinoma. Cancer 1999;85:2119–23.

43. Oizumi H, Matsuda T, Fukase K, et al. Endoscopic resection for early gastric cancer: the actual procedure and clinical evaluation. Stomach and Intestine 1991;85:2119–23.

44. Fukii K, Okajima K, Isozaki H, et al. A clinicopathological study on the indications of limited surgery for submucosal gastric cancer. Japan Journal of Gastroenterology Surgery 1998;31:2055–62.

45. Hirasawa T, Gotoda T, Miyata S, et al. Incidence of lymph node metastasis and the feasibility of endoscopic resection for undifferentiated-type early gastric cancer. Gastric Cancer 2009;12(3):148–52.

46. Kojima T, Parra-Blanco A, Takahashi H, et al. Outcome of endoscopic mucosal resection for early gastric cancer: review of the Japanese literature. Gastrointest Endosc 1998;48(5):550–4 [discussion: 554–5].

47. Uedo N, Iishi H, Tatsuta M, et al. Longterm outcomes after endoscopic mucosal resection for early gastric cancer. Gastric Cancer 2006;9(2):88–92.

48. Choi KS, Jung HY, Choi KD, et al. EMR versus gastrectomy for intramucosal gastric cancer: comparison of long-term outcomes. Gastrointest Endosc 2011;73(5):942–8.

49. Gotoda T, Iwasaki M, Kusano C, et al. Endoscopic resection of early gastric cancer treated by guideline and expanded National Cancer Centre criteria. Br J Surg 2010;97(6):868–71.

50. Etoh T, Katai H, Fukagawa T, et al. Treatment of early gastric cancer in the elderly patient: results of EMR and gastrectomy at a national referral center in Japan. Gastrointest Endosc 2005;62(6):868–71.

51. Kusano C, Iwasaki M, Kaltenbach T, et al. Should elderly patients undergo additional surgery after non-curative endoscopic resection for early gastric cancer? Long-term comparative outcomes. Am J Gastroenterol 2011;106: 1064–9.

52. Nagano H, Ohyama S, Fukunaga T, et al. Two rare cases of node-positive differentiated gastric cancer despite their infiltration to sm1, their small size, and lack of lymphatic invasion into the submucosal layer. Gastric Cancer 2008;11(1): 53–7 [discussion: 57–8].

53. Oya H, Gotoda T, Kinjo T, et al. A case of lymph node metastasis following a curative endoscopic submucosal dissection of an early gastric cancer. Gastric Cancer 2012;15(2):221–5.

54. Chung JW, Jung HY, Choi KD, et al. Extended indication of endoscopic resection for mucosal early gastric cancer: analysis of a single center experience. J Gastroenterol Hepatol 2011;26(5):884–7.

55. Oda I, Gotoda T, Hamanaka H, et al. Endoscopic submucosal dissection for early gastric cancer: technical feasibility, operation time and complications from a large consecutive series. Dig Endosc 2005;17:54–8.

56. Yamamoto S, Uedo N, Ishihara R, et al. Endoscopic submucosal dissection for early gastric cancer performed by supervised residents: assessment of feasibility and learning curve. Endoscopy 2009;41(11):923–8.

57. Fujishiro M, Ono H, Gotoda T, et al. Usefulness of Maalox for detection of the precise bleeding points and confirmation of hemostasis on gastrointestinal hemorrhage. Endoscopy 2001;32:196.

58. Takizawa K, Oda I, Gotoda T, et al. Routine coagulation of visible vessels may prevent delayed bleeding after endoscopic submucosal dissection—an analysis of risk factors. Endoscopy 2008;40(3):179–83.

59. Okano A, Hajiro K, Takakuwa H, et al. Predictors of bleeding after endoscopic mucosal resection of gastric tumors. Gastrointest Endosc 2003;57(6):687–90.

60. Shiba M, Higuchi K, Kadouchi K, et al. Risk factors for bleeding after endoscopic mucosal resection. World J Gastroenterol 2005;11(46):7335–9.

61. Tsunada S, Ogata S, Ohyama T, et al. Endoscopic closure of perforations caused by EMR in the stomach by application of metallic clips. Gastrointest Endosc 2003;57(7):948–51.

62. Minami S, Gotoda T, Ono H, et al. Complete endoscopic closure of gastric perforation induced by endoscopic resection of early gastric cancer using endoclips can prevent surgery (with video). Gastrointest Endosc 2006;63(4): 596–601.

63. Yamamoto H, Kawata H, Sunada K, et al. Success rate of curative endoscopic mucosal resection with circumferential mucosal incision assisted by submucosal injection of sodium hyaluronate. Gastrointest Endosc 2002; 56(4):507–12.

64. Fujishiro M, Yahagi N, Nakamura M, et al. Successful outcomes of a novel endoscopic treatment for GI tumors: endoscopic submucosal dissection with a mixture of high-molecular-weight hyaluronic acid, glycerin, and sugar. Gastrointest Endosc 2006;63(2):243–9.

65. Fujishiro M, Yahagi N, Kashimura K, et al. Tissue damage of different submucosal injection solutions for EMR. Gastrointest Endosc 2005;62(6):933–42.

66. Ikehara H, Gotoda T, Ono H, et al. Gastric perforation during endoscopic resection for gastric carcinoma and the risk of peritoneal dissemination. Br J Surg 2007;94(8):992–5.

67. Yao K, Nagahama T, Matsui T, et al. Detection and characterization of early gastric cancer for curative endoscopic submucosal dissection. Dig Endosc 2013;25(Suppl 1):44–54.

68. Kakushima N, Fujishiro M, Kodashima S, et al. A learning curve for endoscopic submucosal dissection of gastric epithelial neoplasms. Endoscopy 2006;38(10): 991–5.

69. Gotoda T, Friedland S, Hamanaka H, et al. A learning curve for advanced endoscopic resection. Gastrointest Endosc 2005;62(6):866–7.

70. Oda I, Odagaki T, Suzuki H, et al. Learning curve for endoscopic submucosal dissection of early gastric cancer based on trainee experience. Dig Endosc 2012;24(Suppl 1):129–32.

71. Goda K, Fujishiro M, Hirasawa K, et al. How to teach and learn endoscopic submucosal dissection for upper gastrointestinal neoplasm in Japan. Dig Endosc 2012;24:136–42.

72. Hirasawa K, Kokawa A, Oka H, et al. Risk assessment chart for curability of early gastric cancer with endoscopic submucosal dissection. Gastrointest Endosc 2011;74:1268–75.

73. Teoh AY, Chiu PW, Wong SK, et al. Difficulties and outcomes in starting endoscopic submucosal dissection. Surg Endosc 2010;24:1049–54.

74. Parra-Blanco A, Gonzalez N, Arnau MR. Ex vivo and in vivo models for endoscopic submucosal dissection training. Clin Endosc 2012;45:350–7.

75. Parra-Blanco A, Arnau MR, Nicolas-Perez D, et al. Endoscopic submucosal dissection training with pig models in a Western country. World J Gastroenterol 2010;16:2895–900.

76. Berr F, Ponchon T, Neureiter D, et al. Experimental endoscopic submucosal dissection training in a porcine model: learning experience of skilled Western endoscopists. Dig Endosc 2011;23:281–9.
77. Rosch T, Sarbia M, Schumacher B, et al. Attempted endoscopic en bloc resection of mucosal and submucosal tumors using insulated-tip knives: a pilot series. Endoscopy 2004;36:788–801.
78. Dinis-Ribeiro M, Pimentel-Nunes P, Afonso M, et al. A European case series of endoscopic submucosal dissection for gastric superficial lesions. Gastrointest Endosc 2009;69:350–5.
79. Catalano F, Trecca A, Rodella L, et al. The modern treatment of early gastric cancer: our experience in an Italian cohort. Surg Endosc 2009;23:1581–6.
80. Coda S, Trentino P, Antonellis F, et al. A Western single-center experience with endoscopic submucosal dissection for early gastrointestinal cancers. Gastric Cancer 2010;13:258–63.
81. Bialek A, Wiechowska-Kozlowska A, Pertkiewicz J, et al. Endoscopic submucosal dissection for treatment of gastric subepithelial tumors (with video). Gastrointest Endosc 2012;75:276–86.
82. Nonaka S, Saito Y, Takisawa H, et al. Safety of carbon dioxide insufflation for upper gastrointestinal tract endoscopic treatment of patients under deep sedation. Surg Endosc 2010;24:1638–45.
83. Matsui N, Akahoshi K, Nakamura K, et al. Endoscopic submucosal dissection for removal of superficial gastrointestinal neoplasms: a technical review. World J Gastrointest Endosc 2012;4:123–36.
84. Lee WS, Cho JW, Kim YD, et al. Technical issues and new devices of ESD of early gastric cancer. World J Gastroenterol 2011;17:3585–90.
85. Yamamoto H, Yahagi N, Oyama T, et al. Usefulness and safety of 0.4% sodium hyaluronate solution as a submucosal fluid "cushion" in endoscopic resection for gastric neoplasms: a prospective multicenter trial. Gastrointest Endosc 2008;67:830–9.
86. Bacani CJ, Woodward TA, Raimondo M, et al. The safety and efficacy in humans of endoscopic mucosal resection with hydroxypropyl methylcellulose as compared with normal saline. Surg Endosc 2008;22:2401–6.
87. Chan EP, Kaltenbach T, Rouse RV, et al. Potential hazards of submucosal injection of methylene blue. Am J Gastroenterol 2012;107:633–4.
88. Teoh AY, Chiu PW, Hon SF, et al. Ex vivo comparative study using the Endolifter((R)) as a traction device for enhancing submucosal visualization during endoscopic submucosal dissection. Surg Endosc 2012;27:1422–7.
89. Meining A, Schneider A, Roppenecker D, et al. A new instrument for endoscopic submucosal dissection (with videos). Gastrointest Endosc 2013;77:654–7.
90. Von Renteln D, Dulai PS, Pohl H, et al. Endoscopic submucosal dissection with a flexible Maryland dissector: randomized comparison of mesna and saline solution for submucosal injection. Gastrointest Endosc 2011;74:906–11.
91. Akahoshi K, Honda K, Motomura Y, et al. Endoscopic submucosal dissection using a grasping-type scissors forceps for early gastric cancers and adenomas. Dig Endosc 2011;23:24–9.
92. Sakamoto N, Osada T, Shibuya T, et al. Endoscopic submucosal dissection of large colorectal tumors by using a novel spring-action S-O clip for traction (with video). Gastrointest Endosc 2009;69:1370–4.
93. Motohashi O. Two-point fixed endoscopic submucosal dissection in rectal tumor (with video). Gastrointest Endosc 2011;74:1132–6.

94. Gotoda T, Oda I, Tamakawa K, et al. Prospective clinical trial of magnetic-anchor-guided endoscopic submucosal dissection for large early gastric cancer (with videos). Gastrointest Endosc 2009;69:10–5.

95. Yonezawa J, Kaise M, Sumiyama K, et al. A novel double-channel therapeutic endoscope ("R-scope") facilitates endoscopic submucosal dissection of superficial gastric neoplasms. Endoscopy 2006;38:1011–5.

96. Spaun GO, Zheng B, Swanstrom LL. A multitasking platform for natural orifice transluminal endoscopic surgery (NOTES): a benchtop comparison of a new device for flexible endoscopic surgery and a standard dual-channel endoscope. Surg Endosc 2009;23:2720–7.

97. Thompson CC, Ryou M, Soper NJ, et al. Evaluation of a manually driven, multitasking platform for complex endoluminal and natural orifice transluminal endoscopic surgery applications (with video). Gastrointest Endosc 2009;70:121–5.

98. Clayman RV, Box GN, Abraham JB, et al. Rapid communication: transvaginal single-port NOTES nephrectomy: initial laboratory experience. J Endourol 2007;21:640–4.

99. Phee SJ, Kencana AP, Huyunh VA, et al. Design of a master and slave transluminal endoscopic robot for natural orifice transluminal endoscopic surgery. J Mech Eng Sci 2010;224:1495–503.

100. Ho KY, Phee SJ, Shabbir A, et al. Endoscopic submucosal dissection of gastric lesions using a master and slave transluminal endoscopic robot. Gastrointest Endosc 2010;72:593–6.

101. Wang Z, Phee SJ, Lomanto D, et al. Endoscopic submucosal dissection of gastric lesions by using a master and slave transluminal endoscopic robot: an animal survival study. Endoscopy 2012;44:690–4.

102. Phee SJ, Reddy N, Chiu PW, et al. Robot-assisted endoscopic submucosal dissection is effective in treating patients with early-stage gastric neoplasia. Clin Gastroenterol Hepatol 2012;10:1117–21.

103. Nakajima K, Moon JH, Tsutsui S, et al. Esophageal submucosal dissection under steady pressure automatically controlled endoscopy (SPACE): a randomized preclinical trial. Endoscopy 2012;44:1139–48.

Duodenal ESD: Conquering Difficulties

Hironori Yamamoto, MD, PhD*, Yoshimasa Miura, MD

KEYWORDS

- Endoscopic submucosal dissection • Duodenal adenoma • Sodium hialuronate
- Small-caliber-tip transparent hood • Tunneling method • Carcinoma • Therapy

KEY POINTS

- Duodenal endoscopic submucosal dissection (ESD) is technically difficult due to insufficient mucosal elevation and poor mucosal contraction.
- In duodenal ESD, abundant blood vessels in the submucosal layer and thin muscle layer pose a serious risk of bleeding and perforation.
- Selection of ESD in the duodenum should be made cautiously with full consideration of difficulties and risks.
- Minimize thermal injury to the muscle layer to avoid delayed perforation.
- Tunneling method with an ST hood is recommended in duodenal ESD.

 Video of endoscopic submucosal dissection for early duodenal cancer accompanies this article

INTRODUCTION

Endoscopic submucosal dissection (ESD) has been recognized as an advanced endoscopic resection technique effective at achieving en bloc resection of superficial neoplastic lesions. En bloc resection of a large superficial gastric neoplasm without resorting to snaring was first reported by Yamamoto and colleagues[1] in 2001. Initial indication of ESD was mainly focused on gastric lesions.[2,3] Since then, its use has gradually spread to other parts of the gastrointestinal (GI) tract, including the esophagus and colorectum.[4–7] However, duodenal ESD is still considered a difficult procedure with a high risk. Even in Japan, where ESD was developed, duodenal ESD is performed only in a small number of institutions by endoscopists who possess advanced skill and experience in ESD.

Funding sources: Dr H. Yamamoto: Fujifilm Research Fund, Fujifilm. Dr Y. Miura: None.
Conflict of Interest: Dr H. Yamamoto: Consultant for Fujifilm Corporation. Dr Y. Miura: None.
Gastroenterology Center, Jichi Medical University, 3311-1 Yakushiji, Shimotsuke, Tochigi 329-0498, Japan
* Corresponding author.
E-mail address: ireef@jichi.ac.jp

Superficial duodenal neoplasms without lymph node metastasis can be cured by endoscopic resection. Although endoscopic mucosal resection of duodenal neoplasms was first described in 1992,[8] it remains a difficult procedure. Technically, duodenal ESD is considered even more difficult. Although several reports of successful ESD for duodenal lesions have been published,[9–16] application of ESD to duodenal lesions should be prudently selected, knowing that the duodenum is the most difficult and risky place for performing ESD in the GI tract.[17]

This article describes ESD techniques applicable to duodenal lesions.

FACTORS OF DIFFICULTY IN DUODENAL ESD
Anatomic Features

The duodenal wall consists of the mucosal, submucosal, proper muscle, and serosal layers, similar to other areas of the GI tract. However, the posterior wall lacks the serosal layer.

The proper muscle layer of the duodenum is very thin and soft. It is even thinner than in the esophagus and colorectum. Therefore, the duodenal wall is prone to perforation by submucosal dissection technique. Just by exposing the muscle layer on the posterior wall, without obvious perforation, insufflation can cause air leak to the retroperitoneal space through the thin muscle layer.

Risk of delayed perforation is also high in the duodenum, probably due to the thin muscle layer and the hazardous effect of duodenal contents (mainly bile and pancreatic juice). Therefore, submucosal dissection should be performed with minimal thermal injury to the muscle layer and by leaving a thin layer of submucosal tissue on the surface of the muscle layer.

The submucosal tissue of the duodenum is coarse compared with that of the esophagus and colorectum. In the duodenal bulb, adequate mucosal elevation by submucosal injection is often difficult to obtain. This is most likely due to the presence of dense Brunner glands, which make dissection difficult.[14]

In the second and third portion of the duodenum, good mucosal protrusion is usually created by submucosal injection with relative ease. However, it quickly disperses after mucosal incision. Therefore, it is difficult to maintain sufficient submucosal thickening during the ESD procedure in the duodenum.

In addition, blood vessels are abundant in the duodenal submucosal layer. Therefore, it is often difficult to control bleeding during submucosal dissection.

The duodenal mucosal layer also has a unique feature different from other parts of the GI tract. In the esophagus, stomach, and colorectum, mucosa shrinks after incision, resulting in the opening of the wound exposing the submucosal layer. However, duodenal mucosa does not shrink after incision. Therefore, it is difficult to expose the submucosal layer after mucosal incision.

In the second portion of the duodenum, there exist the major and minor papillae. Imprudent or accidental injuries to the papilla can cause pancreatitis. Therefore, the major and minor papillae should be identified to clarify their involvement or proximity to the lesion before starting ESD in the second portion of the duodenum.

All the above-mentioned anatomic features of the duodenum make duodenal ESD technically challenging.

Endoscopic Maneuverability

The duodenum is anatomically fixed in the retroperitoneum. However, endoscopic control in the duodenum is often poor, unstable, and sometimes paradoxic, due to free flexure of endoscope shaft in the wide lumen of the stomach. It is difficult for endoscopists to maintain the proper distance between the tip of the endoscope and the duodenal lesion because of poor control of the flexible endoscope. Rotation of the endoscope shaft to the left can easily cause unintentional withdrawal of the endoscope tip.

Selection of ESD in the Duodenum

Selection of ESD in the duodenum should be made cautiously, with full consideration of the above-mentioned difficulties and risks. However, en bloc R0 resection (complete resection with no microscopic residual tumor) achievable with ESD is also appealing in the duodenum. Using ESD, en bloc R0 resection is achievable even for large flat lesions (**Fig. 1**) or lesions with some fibrosis due to minute submucosal invasion or biopsy scars (**Fig. 2**). Recurrent lesions after piecemeal endoscopic mucosal resection could

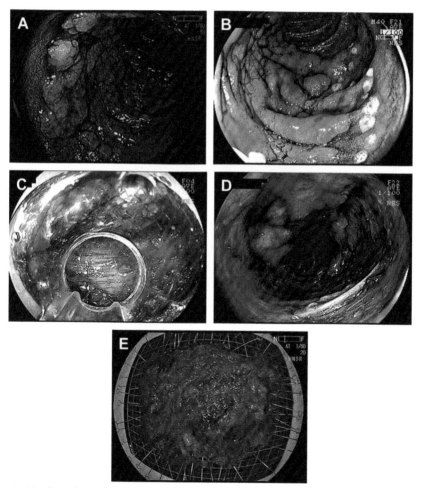

Fig. 1. ESD for a large flat lesion in the second portion of the duodenum. (*A*) Endoscopic view of the large lesion (chromoendoscopy using indigo carmine spray). (*B*) Marking placement around the lesion. (*C*) ESD procedure. (*D*) A large mucosal defect after ESD. (*E*) En bloc resection of the lesion. Pathologic examination of the 91 mm specimen showed well differentiated adenocarcinoma with adenomatous component. Submucosal invasion (−), vessel involvement (−).

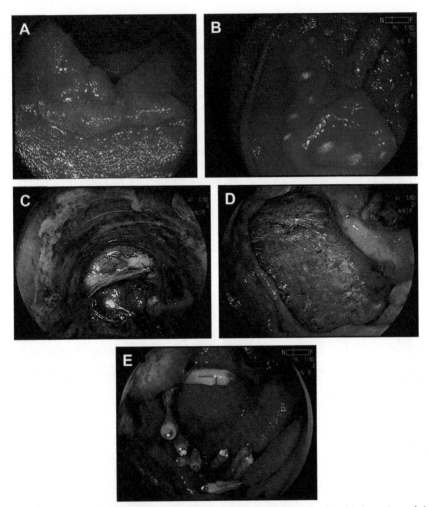

Fig. 2. ESD for a 25 mm flat lesion (adenoma) with a biopsy scar in the third portion of the duodenum. (*A*) Endoscopic view of the IIa lesion. It has a biopsy scar with fold convergence at the center of the lesion suggesting significant submucosal fibrosis. (*B*) Marking placement around the lesion. (*C*) Submucosal endoscopy using an ST hood (tunneling method). (*D*) The mucosal defect after ESD. (*E*) The mucosal defect was closed with clips.

make endoscopic resection even more difficult. Surgical resection procedures for duodenal lesions are complicated and invasive. As long as the procedure is performed reliably and safely, ESD is beneficial for patients, even in the duodenum.

RECOMMENDED TECHNIQUES IN DUODENAL ESD
How to Overcome the Difficulties

For success of ESD, good control of bleeding and selection of a good dissection level (deep enough but not too close to the proper muscle layer; about one-third of submucosa from the muscle layer) in the submucosal layer with minimum tissue damage are important (Video 1). To achieve these goals, submucosal thickening should be maintained and dissection of the submucosal tissue should be performed under clear endoscopic visualization.

Injection Solution

It is particularly important to select a long-lasting injection solution for duodenal ESD. A 0.4% sodium hyaluronate solution (MucoUp, Johnson and Johnson, Tokyo, Japan) is often used in Japan. Sodium hyaluronate is a viscous substance with a high molecular weight that can create a long-lasting mucosal protrusion with submucosal injection.[18] Despite its high viscosity, this isotonic solution causes no damage to the injected tissue.

For submucosal injection of sodium hyaluronate, a 25-gauge needle of a high-flow type with a large luminal inner catheter (Disposable injector 1857, Top, Tokyo, Japan) and a small-caliber syringe such as a 5 mL syringe with a lock should be used to avoid excessive flow resistance in injection.

Preinjection of normal saline into the submucosal layer is useful for avoiding inappropriate injection of sodium hyaluronate into the muscle layer. A small amount of indigo carmine dye (0.004%) and epinephrine (0.001%) in the sodium hyaluronate solution allow the injected area to be distinguished from the noninjected area and reduces the risk of bleeding during ESD.

Transparent Hood and Dissection Technique

To maintain adequate thickening of the submucosal layer in the duodenum, submucosal injection alone is not good enough, even with sodium hyaluronate solution. In this circumstance, the tunneling method using a transparent hood is useful.[19] Once the tip of the endoscope with a transparent hood is inserted into the submucosal layer, mechanical stretching of the submucosal tissue can be obtained by the tip of the transparent hood. By making a submucosal tunnel, the endoscope tip is stabilized to allow precise control of the knife for dissection. With precise control of the knife and a good safety margin obtained by the stretching of the submucosal tissue, selection of a good level of dissection becomes feasible. Adjusting the approach angle of the knife so it is tangential to the wall also is easy with this method. An adjusting force with the endoscope tip can be applied in either direction by pushing the mucosa up or pushing the muscle wall down with the tip of the hood.

A small-caliber-tip transparent hood (ST hood)[4] is particularly useful for the tunneling method in duodenal ESD. An ST hood has a tapered tip with a small diameter at the tip of the hood (**Fig. 3**) that makes the opening of the mucosal incision easier even in the duodenum.

To enter the tip of the hood into the submucosal layer, enough opening of the mucosal incision with additional submucosal dissection at the edge of the lesion is important. After making a mucosal incision with adequate elevation of the mucosa with submucosal injection, additional submucosal dissection should be made with the tip of a knife. At this initial submucosal dissection, the dissection level should be just below the mucosal layer, keeping enough distance from the muscle layer. At this initial stage, the dissection is still under normal mucosa around the neoplastic lesion. Therefore, it is not necessary to dissect at a deeper level close to the muscle layer. The sheath of short needle-type knives, such as a flush knife (1.5 mm; DK2618JN15, Fujifilm Corp, Tokyo, Japan) or a dual knife (KD-650L/Q, Olympus Corp, Tokyo, Japan), can be used to open the mucosal incision.

Mucosal incision should be partial in the entire circumference of the lesion. Circumferential mucosal incision at the beginning of ESD should be avoided to prevent quick dispersion of submucosal injections.

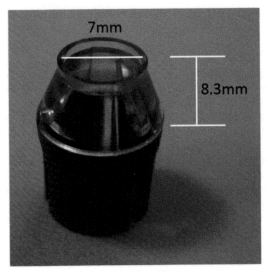

Fig. 3. Small-caliber-tip transparent hood (ST hood).

After mucosal incision and some additional submucosal dissection, the mucosal incision is opened with the tip of the ST hood. The incised mucosa should be gently lifted with the tip of the hood. Forceful push of the tip of the hood should be avoided. With gentle opening of the incision with the hood, submucosal tissue becomes clearly visualized (**Fig. 4**). Submucosal dissection at a desired level can be performed safely under clear visualization of the submucosa.

ESD Knives

A short needle-type knife, such as a flush knife or dual knife, is suitable for duodenal ESD. A ball-tip 1.5 mm flush knife or a 1.5 mm dual knife is the preferred choice in most

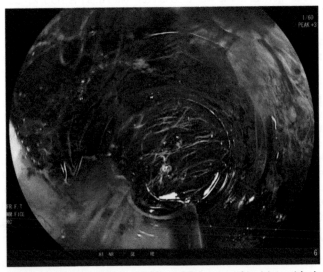

Fig. 4. Submucosal tissue visualized by opening of the mucosal incision with the tip of an ST hood.

cases. However, in difficult situations with fibrosis or an undesirable approaching angle, application of a hook knife (KD 620LR; Olympus Corp, Tokyo, Japan) is recommended. With a hook knife, submucosal tissue can be selectively hooked with the tip of the knife to pull the tissue away from the muscle layer, avoiding muscle injury during application of electricity for cutting.

Hemostasis

Control of bleeding during the procedure is a key factor in successful ESD in the duodenum. Bleeding from abundant blood vessels in the submucosal layer is often caused by submucosal incision performed in a blind fashion. Significant bleeding during submucosal dissection can stain the submucosal tissue red with blood that makes the recognition of blood vessels even more difficult. Therefore, it is important to recognize the blood vessels and coagulate them before cutting. The ST hood enables clear observation of submucosal blood vessels by opening the mucosal incision with its tip.

Small blood vessels can be coagulated with a knife using coagulation mode. For larger vessels, however, coagulation with hemostatic forceps is needed. Hemostatic forceps should be slightly pulled away from the muscle layer before coagulation to prevent electrical injury of the thin muscle layer. In case of bleeding, the bleeding vessel should be grasped with a hemostatic forceps and treated with soft coagulation.

Bipolar hemostatic forceps might be a better choice in the duodenum because deep thermal injuries to the muscle layer can be avoided with bipolar devices.[20]

Stabilization of Endoscopic Maneuver

General anesthesia

In cases with unstable endoscopic control, restlessness of patients with inadequate sedation makes the procedure very difficult or even impossible. In such cases, general anesthesia is recommended to stabilize the patient. Control of bleeding is also easier with general anesthesia, probably due to stable control of blood pressure.

Double-balloon endoscope

When lesions are located in the duodenal portion distal to the papilla of Vater and in cases when the endoscope control becomes unstable, the double-balloon endoscope (DBE) is useful to stabilize the control of the endoscope tip. A short-type DBE (EC-450BI5, Fujifilm, Tokyo, Japan) (**Fig. 5**) is suitable for duodenal ESD.

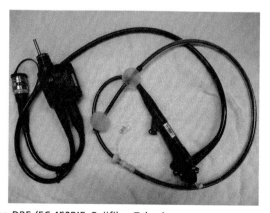

Fig. 5. A short-type DBE (EC-450BI5, Fujifilm, Tokyo).

ESD for lesions involving the papilla of Vater

ESD for lesions involving the papilla of Vater is even more challenging (**Fig. 6**).[21] Mucosal incision at the proximal side should be made with enough distance (about 10 mm) from the papilla of Vater to enable entrance to the submucosal layer with

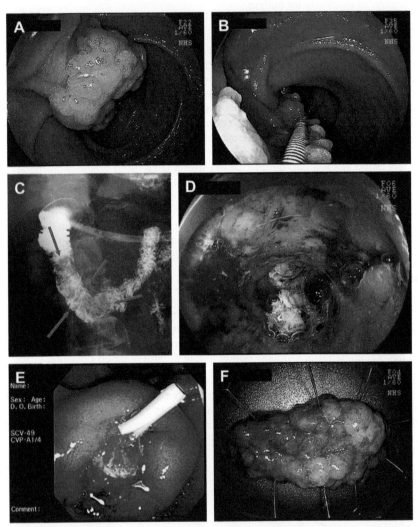

Fig. 6. ESD for a large lesion involving the papilla of Vater. (*A*) Endoscopic image of the large elevated lesion in the second portion of the duodenum. (*B*) Endoscopic view of the lateral side of the lesion. (*C*) Hypotonic duodenography image of the lesion. An elevated lesion (*red arrows*) with granular surface, approximately 6 cm in diameter, was noted from the descending part to the horizontal part of the duodenum. (*D*) Endoscopic image obtained during ESD. The biliary and pancreatic ducts were cut with a needle-knife under direct visualization. (*E*) Endoscopic image obtained just after ESD. A 5F pancreatic-duct stent was inserted into the pancreatic duct. (*F*) Macroscopic image of the resected specimen. The entire lesion was resected in one piece. (*From* Fukushima H, Yamamoto H, Nakano H, et al. Complete en bloc resection of a large ampullary adenoma with a focal adenocarcinoma by using endoscopic submucosal dissection (with video). Gastrointest Endosc 2009;70:592–5; with permission.)

the tip of the ST hood before reaching the papilla. The biliary and pancreatic ducts are visually perceptible in the submucosal layer by continuing the submucosal dissection toward the papilla. The ducts can be cut with a needle-type ESD knife under direct visualization. However, dissection levels tend to become shallow at the papilla. In such cases, a snare ampullectomy can be added after completion of ESD.

A pancreatic duct stent or an endoscopic nasopancreatic drainage (ENPD) tube should be placed to prevent the development of pancreatitis.

How to avoid delayed perforation

The most important factor in avoiding delayed perforation is prevention of thermal injuries to the thin muscle layer. It can be achieved by keeping a safe distance from the muscle layer during submucosal dissection, with the maintenance of its thickness using the above-mentioned injections and techniques.

To avoid the hazardous effects of duodenal content, closure of the mucosal defect with clip placements would be effective (see **Fig. 2**E). When closure of the defect is technically impossible due to the size or location of the defect, placement of an ENPD tube should be considered.

Proton pump inhibitor should be used for ESD in the duodenal bulb. However, its use is controversial for duodenal ESD in the second and third portion of the duodenum. Synthetic protease inhibitors such as nafamostat mesylate could be useful to reduce the hazardous effect of duodenal content by prohibiting the activity of pancreatic enzymes.

It would be prudent to make the fasting period a few days longer in duodenal ESD than other ESDs.

SUMMARY

Duodenal ESD is feasible using proper techniques and instruments. It provides complete en bloc resections with a minimum risk of residual lesions and/or recurrence, in addition to accurate pathologic assessment of the deep and lateral margins of the resected lesions. However, because of the significant technical difficulties and serious risk of complications, duodenal ESD should be performed only in selected patients by sufficiently skilled endoscopists with enough experience with ESD in the stomach, the esophagus, and the colorectum.

SUPPLEMENTARY DATA

Video related to this article can be found online at http://dx.doi.org/10.1016/j.giec.2013.11.007.

REFERENCES

1. Yamamoto H, Sekine Y, Higashizawa T, et al. Successful en bloc resection of a large superficial gastric cancer by using sodium hyaluronate and electrocautery incision forceps. Gastrointest Endosc 2001;54:629–32.
2. Miyamoto S, Muto M, Hamamoto Y, et al. A new technique for endoscopic mucosal resection with an insulated-tip electrosurgical knife improves the completeness of resection of intramucosal gastric neoplasms. Gastrointest Endosc 2002;55:576–81.
3. Yamamoto H, Kawata H, Sunada K, et al. Success rate of curative endoscopic mucosal resection with circumferential mucosal incision assisted by submucosal injection of sodium hyaluronate. Gastrointest Endosc 2002;56:507–12.

4. Yamamoto H, Kawata H, Sunada K, et al. Successful en-bloc resection of large superficial tumors in the stomach and colon using sodium hyaluronate and small-caliber-tip transparent hood. Endoscopy 2003;35:690–4.

5. Oyama T, Tomori A, Hotta K, et al. Endoscopic submucosal dissection of early esophageal cancer. Clin Gastroenterol Hepatol 2005;3:S67–70.

6. Fujishiro M, Yahagi N, Kakushima N, et al. Endoscopic submucosal dissection of esophageal squamous cell neoplasms. Clin Gastroenterol Hepatol 2006;4: 688–94.

7. Yamamoto H, Yahagi N, Oyama T. Mucosectomy in the colon with endoscopic submucosal dissection. Endoscopy 2005;37:764–8.

8. Obata S, Suenaga M, Araki K, et al. Use of strip biopsy in a case of early duodenal cancer. Endoscopy 1992;24:232–4.

9. Ohba R, Otaka M, Jin M, et al. Large Brunner's gland hyperplasia treated with modified endoscopic submucosal dissection. Dig Dis Sci 2007;52:170–2.

10. Honda T, Yamamoto H, Osawa H, et al. Endoscopic submucosal dissection for superficial duodenal neoplasms. Dig Endosc 2009;21:270–4.

11. Takahashi T, Ando T, Kabeshima Y, et al. Borderline cases between benignancy and malignancy of the duodenum diagnosed successfully by endoscopic submucosal dissection. Scand J Gastroenterol 2009;44:1377–83.

12. Chiu PW, Teoh AY, Ng EK. A case of nonampullary duodenal adenoma treated by endoscopic submucosal dissection (with video). Gastrointest Endosc 2010;71: 1328–9.

13. Shinoda M, Makino A, Wada M, et al. Successful endoscopic submucosal dissection for mucosal cancer of the duodenum. Dig Endosc 2010;22:49–52.

14. Jung JH, Choi KD, Ahn JY, et al. Endoscopic submucosal dissection for sessile, nonampullary duodenal adenomas. Endoscopy 2013;45:133–5.

15. Maruoka D, Arai M, Kishimoto T, et al. Clinical outcomes of endoscopic resection for nonampullary duodenal high-grade dysplasia and intramucosal carcinoma. Endoscopy 2013;45:138–41.

16. Matsumoto S, Miyatani H, Yoshida Y. Endoscopic submucosal dissection for duodenal tumors: a single-center experience. Endoscopy 2013;45:136–7.

17. Bourke MJ. Endoscopic resection in the duodenum: current limitations and future directions. Endoscopy 2013;45:127–32.

18. Yamamoto H, Yube T, Isoda N, et al. A novel method of endoscopic mucosal resection using sodium hyaluronate. Gastrointest Endosc 1999;50:251–6.

19. Yamamoto H. Endoscopic submucosal dissection for colorectal tumors. Front Gastrointest Res 2010;27:287–95.

20. Kataoka M, Kawai T, Yagi K, et al. Clinical evaluation of emergency endoscopic hemostasis with bipolar forceps in non-variceal upper gastrointestinal bleeding. Dig Endosc 2010;22:151–5.

21. Fukushima H, Yamamoto H, Nakano H, et al. Complete en bloc resection of a large ampullary adenoma with a focal adenocarcinoma by using endoscopic submucosal dissection (with video). Gastrointest Endosc 2009;70:592–5.

Colorectal ESD
Current Indications and Latest Technical Advances

Yutaka Saito, MD, PhD*, Taku Sakamoto, MD,
Takeshi Nakajima, MD, PhD, Takahisa Matsuda, MD, PhD

KEYWORDS

- Endoscopic submucosal dissection (ESD) • Endoscopic mucosal resection (EMR)
- Endoscopic piecemeal mucosal resection (EPMR) • Colorectum
- Laterally spreading tumor granular type (LST-G)
- Laterally spreading tumor non-granular type (LST-NG)

KEY POINTS

- Endoscopic submucosal dissection (ESD) is a safe and effective procedure for treating colorectal laterally spreading tumors nongranular type (LST-NGs) larger than 20 mm, laterally spreading tumors granular type (LST-Gs) larger than 30 mm, 0-IIc lesions larger than 20 mm, intramucosal tumors with nonlifting sign, and large sessile lesions, which are all difficult to resect en bloc using conventional EMR, providing a higher en bloc resection rate as well as being less invasive than surgery.
- Establishment of a systematic training program for technically more difficult colorectal ESD in addition to further development and refinement of ESD-related instruments, devices, equipment, and injection solutions will help facilitate increased use of colorectal ESD throughout the world.

INTRODUCTION

Surgery had been the only available treatment for large colorectal tumors, even those detected at an early stage. In Japan, endoscopic mucosal resection (EMR)[1–5] is indicated for the treatment of colorectal adenomas, and intramucosal and submucosal superficial (SM1; invasion <1000 μm from the muscularis mucosae) cancers because of the negligible risk of lymph node (LN) metastasis[6] and excellent clinical outcome results.[2–4]

The endoscopic submucosal dissection (ESD) procedure is accepted as a standard minimally invasive treatment for early gastric and esophageal cancers in Japan.[7,8] Yamamoto and colleagues[9] and Fujishiro, Yahagi and colleagues and colleagues[10]

Endoscopy Division, National Cancer Center Hospital, 5-1-1 Tsukiji, Chuo-ku, Tokyo 104-0045, Japan
* Corresponding author.
E-mail address: ytsaito@ncc.go.jp

Gastrointest Endoscopy Clin N Am 24 (2014) 245–255
http://dx.doi.org/10.1016/j.giec.2013.11.005
1052-5157/14/$ – see front matter © 2014 Elsevier Inc. All rights reserved.

first started performing colorectal ESDs in the early 2000s, but such procedures were being conducted by only a limited number of specialists. Because of the widespread acceptance of gastric and esophageal ESDs, the number of medical facilities that perform colorectal ESDs has been growing, and the effectiveness of colorectal ESD has been increasingly reported in recent years.[11–15]

Until the spring of 2012, colorectal ESDs had been performed in Japan in accordance with advanced medical treatment system No. 78 approved by the Japanese Ministry of Health, Labor, and Welfare in 2009, which distinguishes colorectal ESD from gastric and esophageal ESDs because of its greater technical difficulty.[15] The indications for colorectal ESD under this system were defined as (1) early colorectal cancers larger than 20 mm difficult to treat en bloc by EMR; and (2) adenomas with nonlifting sign or residual tumors larger than 10 mm difficult to treat by EMR.[16]

All candidate lesions for ESD had to be confirmed as being an intramucosal tumor using magnification colonoscopy[16–18] or endoscopic ultrasonography (EUS) before performing the procedure. More than 150 institutions had started performing colorectal ESDs in accordance with the advanced medical treatment system by using recent improvements in ESD-related instruments and devices, as well as various other technical innovations. In fact, a total of 3006 colorectal ESDs were performed in 143 institutions during a recent 1-year period using this advanced medical treatment system. Based on the reported excellent clinical results of colorectal ESDs in Japan, the Japanese health care insurance system has approved colorectal ESD for coverage and set the cost at 183,700 Japanese yen, which is approximately 3 times higher than the cost for conventional EMR. However, most patients younger than 75 years receive a 70% reduction in the treatment cost under the universal health insurance system in Japan.[15]

INDICATIONS FOR COLORECTAL ESD

The indications for colorectal ESD approved by the Japanese government's medical insurance system are colorectal adenomas and cancers with a maximum tumor size of 2 to 5 cm, taking into account the procedure's technical standardization and safety throughout Japan at the present time (**Table 1**).

Based on our previous clinicopathological analyses of laterally spreading tumors (LSTs),[5,16] LST nongranular type (LST-NGs) lesions have a higher rate of submucosal (SM) invasion, which can be difficult to predict endoscopically. Approximately 30% of LST-NGs with SM invasion are multifocal and such invasions are primarily SM superficial (SM1), which is especially difficult to predict before endoscopic treatment. LST-granular type (LST-Gs) lesions have a lower rate of SM invasion and most such invasions are found under the largest nodule or depression and are easier to predict endoscopically.[5,17] LST-Gs larger than 20 mm can be treated by planning endoscopic piecemeal mucosal resection (EPMR) rather than ESD, with the area having the largest nodule resected first before resection of the remaining tumor. LST-Gs larger than 30 mm are possible candidates for ESD, however, because they have a higher SM invasion rate and are more difficult to treat even by EPMR. Consequently, they are treated by either EPMR or ESD depending on the individual endoscopist's judgment.

The 0-IIc lesions larger than 20 mm, intramucosal tumors with nonlifting sign, and large sessile lesions, all of which are difficult to resect en bloc by conventional EMR, are also potential candidates for colorectal ESD.

Residual and recurrent tumors can be treated by ESD depending on the circumstances; however, such lesions usually involve severe fibrosis so they are not good candidates, except in the lower rectum, where the risk of perforation is very low.[17]

Table 1
Indications for colorectal ESD at National Cancer Center Hospital

Noninvasive Pattern Should be Diagnosed by Chromo-magnification Colonoscopy				
Tumor size, mm	<10	≥10–<20	≥20–<30	≥30
0-IIa, IIc, IIa + IIc (LST-NG)[a]	EMR	EMR	ESD	ESD
0-Is + IIa (LST-G)[b]	EMR	EMR	EMR	ESD
0-Is (villous)[c]	EMR	EMR	EMR	ESD
Intramucosal tumor with nonlifting sign[d]	EMR	EMR/ESD	ESD	ESD
Rectal carcinoid tumor[e]	EMR	ESD/Surgery	Surgery	Surgery

Noninvasive pattern diagnosed by chromo-magnification colonoscopy.

Abbreviations: EMR, endoscopic mucosal resection; EPMR, endoscopic piecemeal mucosal resection; ESD, endoscopic submucosal dissection; LST-G, laterally spreading tumor granular type; LST-NG, laterally spreading tumor nongranular type.

[a] 0-IIa, IIc, IIa + IIc (LST-NGs) >20 mm.
[b] 0-Is + IIa (LST-G) >30 mm.
[c] 0-Is (villous) >30 mm.
[d] Intramucosal tumors with nonlifting sign that are difficult to resect en bloc by conventional EMR. Residual and recurrent tumors can be treated by ESD depending on the circumstances; however, such lesions usually involve severe fibrosis so they are not good candidates except in the lower rectum where the perforation risk is very low.
[e] Rectal carcinoid tumors <1 cm in diameter can be treated by endoscopic submucosal resection using a ligation device simply, safely, and effectively, so not an indication for ESD.

Rectal carcinoid tumors smaller than 1 cm in diameter can be treated by endoscopic submucosal resection using a ligation device safely, effectively, and easily, so are not an indication for ESD.[18,19]

ESTIMATING DEPTH OF INVASION

A noninvasive pattern[20,21] and Sano Type II or IIIA capillary pattern (**Fig. 1**C)[22,23] should be confirmed in each lesion (see **Fig. 1**A–D), indicating that the lesion is suitable for EMR or ESD with the estimated invasion depth being less than SM1. No biopsies are recommended before ESD because they can cause fibrosis and may interfere with SM lifting.

ESD PROCEDURE AT NATIONAL CANCER CENTER HOSPITAL
Materials

Endoscope system
The endoscope system included a water jet endoscope (PCF-Q260JI and GIF-Q260J; Olympus Medical Systems Corp, Tokyo, Japan) with a water jet pump system (OFP1; Olympus Medical Systems Corp) (see **Fig. 1**).

ESD knives
ESD knives included a ball-tip bipolar needle knife with water jet function (Jet B-knife) (XEMEX Co, Tokyo, Japan) and a newly developed insulation-tipped electrosurgical knife (IT knife nano) (KD-612Q; Olympus Optical Co, Tokyo, Japan), in which the insulation-tip is smaller and the short-blade is designed as a small disk to reduce the burning effect on the muscle layer.

Distal attachment
Distal attachment was an ST hood short-type (DH-28GR and 29CR; Fujifilm Medical Co, Tokyo, Japan).

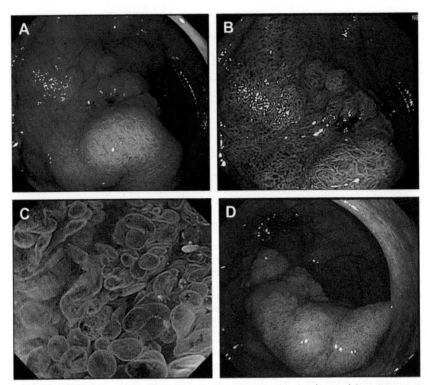

Fig. 1. ESD procedure. (*A, B*) LST-G–type lesion 100 mm in size located in upper rectum (white light image in *A* and narrow band imaging (NBI) image in *B*). (*C*) A noninvasive Sano Type IIIA capillary pattern was confirmed in this lesion, indicating that the lesion was suitable for ESD with the estimated invasion depth being less than SM1. No biopsies were performed before ESD because they could cause fibrosis and could interfere with SM lifting. (*D*) Lesion margins delineated before ESD using 0.4% indigo-carmine dye spraying.

Carbon dioxide regulator

The CO_2 regulator was a UCR (Olympus Medical Systems) or Gas Regulator, Crown (Model FR-IIS-P; Yutaka Engineering, Tokyo, Japan).[12,24]

Bipolar hemostatic forceps

The bipolar hemostatic forceps used were the HemoStat-Y forceps (H-S2518; Pentax Co, Tokyo, Japan).

Submucosal injection solution

Mixtures of 2 solutions were prepared before ESD to create a longer-lasting SM fluid cushion.

> Solution 1: Indigo-carmine dye (2 mL of 1%) and epinephrine (1 mL of 0.1%) were mixed with 200 mL Glyceol (Glyceol, Chugai Pharmaceutical Co, Tokyo, Japan)[25] (10% glycerin and 5% fructose) in a container, and the solution was then drawn into a 5-mL disposable syringe.
>
> Solution 2: MucoUp (MucoUp, Seikakagu Co, Tokyo, Japan)[9] was drawn into another 5-mL syringe.

During the actual ESD procedure, a small amount of solution 1 was injected into the SM layer first to confirm the appropriate SM layer elevation and then solution 2 was injected into the properly elevated SM layer. Finally, a small amount of solution 1 was injected again to flush any residual amount of solution 2.

Electrosurgical generators

The electrosurgical generators were the VIO300D (**Table 2**) (ERBE, Tubingen, Germany) and ESG100 (Olympus Medical Co, Tokyo, Japan).

Colorectal ESD Procedures

The procedures were primarily performed using a Jet B-knife and an IT knife nano[21] with CO_2 insufflation[12,24] instead of air insufflation to reduce patient discomfort (see **Fig. 1**; **Fig. 2**). A short-type ST hood (see **Fig. 2**A, B) was used from the start of each colorectal ESD to creep into the narrow SM layer more easily and provide countertraction for the resected specimen.

After the colorectal ESD was completed, routine colonoscopic review to detect any possible perforation or exposed vessels was conducted (see **Fig. 2**C), and minimum coagulation was performed using the Hemostat-Y forceps on nonbleeding visible thick vessels to prevent postoperative bleeding. The resected specimen was stretched and fixed to a board using small pins (see **Fig. 2**D).

CLINICAL OUTCOMES OF ESDS AT NATIONAL CANCER CENTER HOSPITAL

The en bloc resection rate was 91% and the curative resection rate was 87% for 900 ESDs (**Table 3**). There were a total of 687 (76%) carcinomas; among them, 117 cases (13%) were diagnosed as SM deep and/or positive for lympho-vascular invasion, and additional surgery was recommended for most such noncurative cases. The median procedure time was 60 minutes with a mean of 100 minutes and the mean size of resected specimens was 40 mm (range 20–150 mm). The postoperative bleeding rate for colorectal ESD was 1.7% (15/900) and the perforation rate was 2.7% (24/900), but only one immediate and one delayed perforation required emergency surgery.

In our previously reported prospective multicenter study, multivariate analysis revealed that large tumor size (≥50 mm) and a lower experience level in which fewer

Table 2
The setting of VIO300D for colorectal endoscopic submucosal dissection at National Cancer Center Hospital

Device	Procedure	VIO300D
Jet B-knife	Mucosal cutting	Drycut effect 3, 80 W
	Submucosal dissection	Swift coagulation. Effect 2, 40 W
	Coagulation	Forced coagulation. Effect 2, 40 W
IT knife nano	Mucosal cutting	Drycut effect 3, 80 W
	Submucosal dissection	Swift coagulation. Effect 2, 40 W
	Coagulation	Forced coagulation. Effect 2, 40 W
Hemostat-Y	Coagulation	Bipolar soft effect 4, 25 W

The setting of VIO300D for colorectal endoscopic submucosal dissection at National Cancer Center Hospital.
Jet B-knife and IT knife nano
 Drycut mode (80 W, effect 3) for marginal resection.
 Forced coagulation mode or swift coagulation mode of 40 W, effect 2 for SM dissection.
Hemostat-Y
Bipolar soft mode (25 W, effect 4).

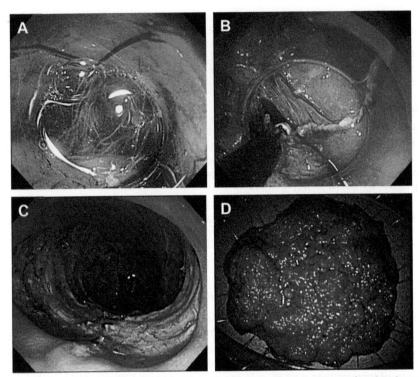

Fig. 2. ESD procedure. (*A*) An ST hood short-type was used from the start of each colorectal ESD to creep into the narrow SM layer more easily and provide countertraction for the resected specimen. Thick vessels could be visualized clearly, so precoagulation was necessary using Hemostat-Y before SM dissection. (*B*) Following injection of glycerol and sodium hyaluronate acid solution into the SM layer, SM dissection of lesion was performed by using the IT knife nano. (*C*) Ulcer bed after successful en bloc resection completed. (*D*) Resected specimen 100 × 80 mm in diameter with tumor-free margins. Histology revealed an intramucosal cancer and curative R0 resection was completed.

Table 3
Clinical results of colorectal ESDs at National Cancer Center Hospital

Years	2004–2012
No. of endoscopic submucosal dissections (n)	900
Tumor location Rectum/Total n (%)	238/900 (26%)
Age, y mean±SD	66 ± 10
Mean tumor size, mm mean±SD	37 ± 18
Mean procedure time, min (median) mean±SD, min. (median)	100 ± 70 (60)
En-bloc resections n/total (%)	728/900 (91%)
Snare use n/total (%)	203/900 (23%)
Cancer %	76%
Curative resections n/total (%)	783/900 (87%)
Perforations n (%)	24 (2.7%)
Delayed bleeding cases n (%)	15 (1.7%)

than 50 ESDs were performed were independent factors for a significantly increased risk of complications.[26]

TECHNICAL PROGRESS OF COLORECTAL ESD

Until recently, colorectal ESDs had been performed mainly in Japan,[9–15,24,26–29] because of the procedure's technical difficulty and because ESD is most frequently used to treat early gastric cancer, which is much more common in Japan than in Western countries,[30] although some trained endoscopists have started to do colorectal ESDs in other Asian countries, including South Korea,[15,31,32] as well as in Europe[33,34] and the United States.[35] One of our Japanese colleagues, Dr Norio Fukami, is now working in the United States in Colorado, routinely performing many successful ESDs,[36] but there is an issue of the limited availability of dedicated devices and solutions for safer ESD in the United States.

To reduce the perforation rate for colorectal ESD, the use of specialized knives,[7,8,27] distal attachments,[9] and hypertonic solutions (glycerol[25] and MucoUp[9]), which produce longer-lasting and higher SM elevation cushions, are necessary for safer ESDs because of the thinner colonic wall. The Jet B-knife is safer because electric current is limited to the needle, the bipolar system prevents electric current from passing to the muscle layer, and the new water-jet function with which SM injection is possible reduces the need for more frequent device changes.

ESD enables treatment of even recurrent lesions after incomplete endoscopic resections, as well as large colorectal LSTs (>10 cm in diameter), but such ESDs are still challenging even in an expert's hands.[26] It is important, therefore, to examine lesions carefully using chromo-magnification colonoscopy[19,20] and to diagnose them accurately before treatment, to reduce unnecessary noncurative resections of SM deep invasive cancers.[6]

Comparison Between ESD and EMR

The primary advantage of ESD compared with EMR is a higher en bloc resection rate for large colonic tumors that had been treated by surgery previously. Consequently, ESD has a lower recurrence rate compared with EMR (2% vs 14%), providing a better quality of life for patients compared with surgery.[37] Future studies should be designed to compare the clinical outcomes between ESD and surgery rather than between ESD and EMR, because the indications for ESD and EMR are different, as are the relevant tumor characteristics.

In the past, EPMR had been considered a feasible treatment for colorectal LSTs because of a low local recurrence rate for such tumors and repeat endoscopic resection was considered sufficient for most local recurrent tumors in Japan.[37,38] In Western countries, EPMR is still the gold standard treatment for LSTs larger than 20 mm in diameter.[39] In our case series,[37] EPMR also was effective in treating many LST-Gs 20 mm or larger, but 3 cases (1.3%) required surgery after such piecemeal resections, including 2 cases of invasive carcinoma recurrence. Based on our results, EPMR cases for LSTs 30 mm or larger should be considered for ESD or laparoscopic-assisted colorectal (LAC) surgery because of the increased risk of SM invasion and because accurate histologic evaluation is difficult in such cases.[16,37]

COMPARISON OF ESD AND SURGERY

LAC is one of the minimally invasive alternatives to open surgery for colorectal cancers, whereas ESD is another such alternative. Comparative effectiveness data on ESD versus LAC resection of early colorectal cancer has so far been unavailable, although such information would be most enlightening given the considerable differences in the potential benefits and risks between the 2 procedures.

We compared ESD with LAC, therefore, as minimally invasive treatments for early colorectal cancer.[40] This comparison indicated that ESD was safe and provided an excellent prognosis despite different indications for ESD and LAC. In terms of the length of hospital stay and time to oral intake after the procedures, both periods were shorter for the ESD group than for the LAC group. ESD and LAC have quite different indications, however, so if the primary indications are a noninvasive colorectal lesion diagnosed preoperatively as intramucosal to SM1 (<1000 μm), the patient's quality of life following treatment for such an early colorectal cancer would probably be better with ESD.[40,41]

Although there have been some cases requiring additional surgical resection after endoscopic resection for SM invasive cancer,[41] colorectal ESD has succeeded in reducing avoidable surgery for mucosal carcinomas and improving the overall quality of life for most patients.

For rectal cancer treatment, however, a longer procedure time is required for LAC compared with ESD, and transanal resection is more invasive than ESD with a significantly higher recurrence rate.[42,43] Accordingly, ESD is the preferred choice for noninvasive rectal cancers.

POST-ESD CARE RECOMMENDATIONS

Supported by our comparative data analysis between ESD and EMR, follow-up endoscopy is recommended after 1 year for curative en bloc ESD cases and after 6 months for piecemeal ESD cases, considering local recurrence rates.[37,38] Even for pathologically curative resection cases, computed tomography (CT) or EUS examination is recommended for SM1 and piecemeal resection cases to detect LN metastasis or distant metastasis. Colonoscopy and a CT scan are scheduled every 12 months, whereas carcinoembryonic antigen (CEA) is checked every 6 months for at least 5 years at National Cancer Center Hospital (the authors' institution).

Surgery is recommended for SM2 or deeper invasion and when lymphovascular invasion or poorly differentiated cancer is diagnosed histologically.[6]

ESTABLISHMENT OF SYSTEMATIC TRAINING FOR COLORECTAL ESD

Probst and colleagues[34] reported that ESD performed in the distal colon is feasible with acceptable complication risks in a European setting. They also indicated resection rates were not as high as those reported in Japanese studies, although a clear learning curve was evident from their results.

Establishment of a systematic training program for technically more difficult colorectal ESD, together with further development and refinement of the instruments, devices, equipment, and injection solutions used in the procedure, are encouraged to facilitate increased use of colorectal ESD not only in Japan, but also in the rest of the world, where there is much less clinical experience in using ESD.[44]

SUMMARY

ESD is a safe and effective procedure for treating colorectal LST-NGs larger than 20 mm, LST-Gs larger than 30 mm, 0-IIc lesions larger than 20 mm, intramucosal tumors with nonlifting sign, and large sessile lesions, which are all difficult to resect en bloc using conventional EMR, providing a higher en bloc resection rate, as well as being less invasive than surgery. Establishment of a systematic training program for technically more difficult colorectal ESD in addition to further development and refinement of ESD-related instruments, devices, equipment, and injection solutions will help facilitate increased use of colorectal ESD throughout the world.

REFERENCES

1. Ahmad NA, Kochman ML, Long WB, et al. Efficacy, safety, and clinical outcomes of endoscopic mucosal resection: a study of 101 cases. Gastrointest Endosc 2002;55:390–6.
2. Yokota T, Sugihara K, Yoshida S. Endoscopic mucosal resection for colorectal neoplastic lesions. Dis Colon Rectum 1994;37:1108–11.
3. Soetikno RM, Gotoda T, Nakanishi Y, et al. Endoscopic mucosal resection. Gastrointest Endosc 2003;57:567–79.
4. Saito Y, Fujii T, Kondo H, et al. Endoscopic treatment for laterally spreading tumors in the colon. Endoscopy 2001;33:682–6.
5. Kudo S, Kashida H, Tamura T, et al. Colonoscopic diagnosis and management of nonpolypoid early colorectal cancer. World J Surg 2000;24:1081–90.
6. Kitajima K, Fujimori T, Fujii S, et al. Correlations between lymph node metastasis and depth of submucosal invasion in submucosal invasive colorectal carcinoma: a Japanese collaborative study. J Gastroenterol 2004;39:534–43.
7. Hosokawa K, Yoshida S. Recent advances in endoscopic mucosal resection for early gastric cancer [in Japanese with English abstract]. Jpn J Canc Chemother 1998;25:476–83.
8. Ono H, Kondo H, Gotoda T, et al. Endoscopic mucosal resection for treatment of early gastric cancer. Gut 2001;48:225–9.
9. Yamamoto H, Kawata H, Sunada K, et al. Successful en-bloc resection of large superficial tumors in the stomach and colon using sodium hyaluronate and small-caliber-tip transparent hood. Endoscopy 2003;35:690–4.
10. Fujishiro M, Yahagi N, Kakushima N, et al. Outcomes of endoscopic submucosal dissection for colorectal epithelial neoplasms in 200 consecutive cases. Clin Gastroenterol Hepatol 2007;5:674–7.
11. Saito Y, Emura F, Matsuda T, et al. A new sinker-assisted endoscopic submucosal dissection for colorectal tumors. Gastrointest Endosc 2005;62:297–301.
12. Saito Y, Uraoka T, Matsuda T, et al. A pilot study to assess safety and efficacy of carbon dioxide insufflation during colorectal endoscopic submucosal dissection under conscious sedation. Gastrointest Endosc 2007;65:537–42.
13. Saito Y, Uraoka T, Matsuda T, et al. Endoscopic treatment of large superficial colorectal tumors: a cases series of 200 endoscopic submucosal dissections (with video). Gastrointest Endosc 2007;66:966–73.
14. Yamazaki K, Saito Y, Fukuzawa M. Endoscopic submucosal dissection of a large laterally spreading tumor in the rectum is a minimally invasive treatment. Clin Gastroenterol Hepatol 2008;6:e5–6.
15. Saito Y, Kawano H, Takeuchi Y, et al. Current status of colorectal endoscopic submucosal dissection in Japan and other Asian countries: progressing towards technical standardization. Dig Endosc 2012;24(Suppl 1):67–72.
16. Uraoka T, Saito Y, Matsuda T, et al. Endoscopic indications for endoscopic mucosal resection of laterally spreading tumours in the colorectum. Gut 2006;55:1592–7.
17. Sakamoto T, Saito Y, Matsuda T, et al. Treatment strategy for recurrent or residual colorectal tumors after endoscopic resection. Surg Endosc 2011;25:255–60.
18. Ono A, Fujii T, Saito Y, et al. Endoscopic submucosal resection of rectal carcinoid tumors with a ligation device. Gastrointest Endosc 2003;57:583–7.

19. Mashimo Y, Matsuda T, Uraoka T, et al. Endoscopic submucosal resection with a ligation device is an effective and safe treatment for carcinoid tumors in the lower rectum. J Gastroenterol Hepatol 2008;23:218–21.

20. Fujii T, Hasegawa RT, Saitoh Y, et al. Chromoscopy during colonoscopy. Endoscopy 2001;33:1036–41.

21. Matsuda T, Fujii T, Saito Y, et al. Efficacy of the invasive/non-invasive pattern by magnifying estimate the depth of invasion of early colorectal neoplasms. Am J Gastroenterol 2008;103:2700–6.

22. Sano Y, Ikematsu H, Fu KI, et al. Meshed capillary vessels by use of narrow-band imaging for differential diagnosis of small colorectal polyps. Gastrointest Endosc 2009;69:278–83.

23. Ikematsu H, Matsuda T, Emura F, et al. Efficacy of capillary pattern type IIIA/IIIB by magnifying narrow band imaging for estimating depth of invasion of early colorectal neoplasms. BMC Gastroenterol 2010;10:33.

24. Kikuchi T, Fu KI, Saito Y, et al. Transcutaneous monitoring of partial pressure of carbon dioxide during endoscopic submucosal dissection of early colorectal neoplasia with carbon dioxide insufflation: a prospective study. Surg Endosc 2010;24:2231–5.

25. Uraoka T, Fujii T, Saito Y, et al. Effectiveness of glycerol as a submucosal injection for EMR. Gastrointest Endosc 2005;61:736–40.

26. Saito Y, Uraoka T, Yamaguchi Y, et al. A prospective, multicenter study of 1111 colorectal endoscopic submucosal dissections (with video). Gastrointest Endosc 2010;72:1217–25.

27. Hotta K, Yamaguchi Y, Saito Y, et al. Current opinions for endoscopic submucosal dissection for colorectal tumors from our experiences: indications, technical aspects and complications. Dig Endosc 2012;24(Suppl 1):110–6.

28. Tamegai Y, Saito Y, Masaki N, et al. Endoscopic submucosal dissection: a safe technique for colorectal tumors. Endoscopy 2007;39:418–22.

29. Tanaka S, Oka S, Kaneko I, et al. Endoscopic submucosal dissection for colorectal neoplasia: possibility of standardization. Gastrointest Endosc 2007;66:100–7.

30. Friedland S, Sedehi D, Soetikno R. Colonoscopic polypectomy in anticoagulated patients. World J Gastroenterol 2009;15:1973–6.

31. Lee EJ, Lee JB, Lee SH, et al. Endoscopic submucosal dissection for colorectal tumors-1,000 colorectal ESD cases: one specialized institute's experiences. Surg Endosc 2013;27(1):31–9.

32. Kang KJ, Kim DU, Kim BJ, et al. Endoscopy-based decision is sufficient for predicting completeness in lateral resection margin in colon endoscopic submucosal dissection. Digestion 2012;85:33–9.

33. Hurlstone DP, Atkinson R, Sanders DS, et al. Achieving R0 resection in the colorectum using endoscopic submucosal dissection. Br J Surg 2007;94:1536–42.

34. Probst A, Golger D, Anthuber M, et al. Endoscopic submucosal dissection in large sessile lesions of the rectosigmoid: learning curve in a European center. Endoscopy 2012;44:660–7.

35. Antillon MR, Bartalos CR, Miller ML, et al. En bloc endoscopic submucosal dissection of a 14-cm laterally spreading adenoma of the rectum with involvement to the anal canal: expanding the frontiers of endoscopic surgery (with video). Gastrointest Endosc 2008;67:332–7.

36. Fukami N, Ryu CB, Said S, et al. Prospective, randomized study of conventional versus HybridKnife endoscopic submucosal dissection methods for the esophagus: an animal study. Gastrointest Endosc 2011;73:1246–53.

37. Saito Y, Fukuzawa M, Matsuda T, et al. Clinical outcome of endoscopic submucosal dissection versus endoscopic mucosal resection of large colorectal tumors as determined by curative resection. Surg Endosc 2010;24:343–52.

38. Hotta K, Fujii T, Saito Y, et al. Local recurrence after endoscopic resection of colorectal tumors. Int J Colorectal Dis 2009;24(2):225–30.

39. Moss A, Bourke MJ, Williams SJ, et al. Endoscopic mucosal resection outcomes and prediction of submucosal cancer from advanced colonic mucosal neoplasia. Gastroenterology 2011;140:1909–18.

40. Kiriyama S, Saito Y, Yamamoto S, et al. Comparison of endoscopic submucosal dissection with laparoscopic-assisted colorectal surgery for early-stage colorectal cancer: a retrospective analysis. Endoscopy 2012;44:1024–30.

41. Kobayashi N, Saito Y, Uraoka T, et al. Treatment strategy for laterally spreading tumors in Japan: before and after the introduction of endoscopic submucosal dissection. J Gastroenterol Hepatol 2009;24:1387–92.

42. Kiriyama S, Saito Y, Matsuda T, et al. Comparing endoscopic submucosal dissection with transanal resection for non-invasive rectal tumor: a retrospective study. J Gastroenterol Hepatol 2011;26:1028–33.

43. Park SU, Min YW, Shin JU, et al. Endoscopic submucosal dissection or transanal endoscopic microsurgery for nonpolypoid rectal high grade dysplasia and submucosa-invading rectal cancer. Endoscopy 2012;44:1031–6.

44. Parra-Blanco A, Gonzalez N, Arnau MR. Ex vivo and in vivo models for endoscopic submucosal dissection training. Clin Endosc 2012;45:350–7.

Submucosal Endoscopy
From ESD to POEM and Beyond

Haruhiro Inoue, MD, PhD[a],*, Esperanza Grace Santi, MD, PhD[b],
Manabu Onimaru, MD, PhD[a], Shin-ei Kudo, MD, PhD[a]

KEYWORDS

- Endoscopic mucosal resection • Endoscopic submucosal dissection
- Peroral endoscopic myotomy • Achalasia • Heller myotomy
- Submucosal endoscopic tumor reaction • Submucosal tumor

KEY POINTS

- The development of snare polypectomy with electrocautery opened the door for therapeutic endoscopy in the gastrointestinal tract.
- At present, endoscopic submucosal dissection (ESD) consists of endoscopic microsurgery using a flexible endoscope.
- In both ESD and peroral endoscopic myotomy (POEM) if either the mucosa or the muscle layer are kept intact, neither peritonitis nor mediastinitis may occur, because either the mucosa or the muscle layer acts as a strong barrier.
- POEM is performed under general anesthesia with endotracheal intubation, keeping the patient in the supine position.
- Another major advantage of POEM is the flexibility of myotomy length.

INTRODUCTION

Peroral endoscopic myotomy (POEM)[1] is an evolving minimally invasive endoscopic surgical procedure, with no skin incision, intended for long-term recovery from symptoms of esophageal achalasia. POEM is considered one of the best applications of NOTES (Natural Orifice Transluminal Endoscopic Surgery).[2] The first case was performed on September 8, 2008 at Showa University Northern Yokohama Hospital.[3] Since then more than 390 achalasia cases have been treated with the POEM procedure in this hospital, with no major complications. POEM was developed based on both the already established surgical principles of esophageal myotomy and the

[a] Digestive Disease Center, Showa University Koto-Toyosu Hospital, Yokohama, Japan;
[b] Section of Gastroenterology, Department of Internal Medicine, De La Salle University Medical Center, Manila, Philippines
* Corresponding author.
E-mail address: haruinoue777@yahoo.co.jp

Gastrointest Endoscopy Clin N Am 24 (2014) 257–264
http://dx.doi.org/10.1016/j.giec.2013.12.003
1052-5157/14/$ – see front matter © 2014 Elsevier Inc. All rights reserved.

advanced techniques of endoscopic submucosal dissection (ESD). This article relates how POEM was developed, and its use in practice is reported and discussed. As an extension of the POEM technique, submucosal endoscopic tumor resection is introduced.[4]

ADVANCEMENT IN TECHNOLOGY FROM ENDOSCOPIC MUCOSAL RESECTION/ESD TO POEM

The development of snare polypectomy with electrocautery opened the door for therapeutic endoscopy in the gastrointestinal tract. With less risk of bleeding, snare polypectomy quickly became the standard treatment for polypoid lesions. However, application of snare polypectomy to nonpolypoid lesions was technically difficult and remained unsolved. Endoscopic mucosal resection (EMR) was then developed for resection of flat mucosal lesions. Dehyle and colleagues[5] reported endoscopic resection of mucosa combined with submucosal injection. Submucosal injection creates a mucosal bleb, which is followed by snare resection. Later, EMR using a suction cap (EMR-C) was developed by the authors.[6] EMR-C was then further modified to EMR using a band ligator,[7,8] which accelerated the popularization of the technique. EMR does enable the resection of flat mucosal lesions, but the size of resection is somewhat limited. Large mucosal lesions can be successfully excised in a piecemeal fashion through repeated EMRs, although the resulting specimens are fragmented.[9,10]

To acquire large, one-piece specimens for accurate histopathologic evaluation, the novel method of ESD was developed by Ono.[11] To successfully complete ESD, various basic techniques are used such as submucosal injection, mucosal cutting, submucosal dissection, and hemostasis. ESD currently consists of endoscopic microsurgery using a flexible endoscope. The fundamental techniques used in the POEM procedure (submucosal injection, mucosal incision, submucosal tunneling, and hemostasis) are very similar to those of ESD.

HISTORY OF ACHALASIA TREATMENT

Achalasia (the word itself is a Greek term that means "does not relax") is a chronic benign disease with a subtle onset and symptoms that may progress gradually for years before an exact diagnosis can be made.[12] It is the most common primary motility disorder of the esophagus; however, it occurs rarely, with an annual incidence of approximately 0.03 to 1 per 100,000 per year. Achalasia affects men and women equally and may occur at any age. Despite an increasing understanding of its pathophysiology, the etiology of achalasia remains largely unknown,[13] and all current treatments have different advantages and drawbacks.[14–17]

Therapy has focused mainly on the forced relaxation of the lower esophageal sphincter (LES) by endoscopic or surgical means. As few randomized controlled trials have attempted to determine the optimal strategy, treatment still varies widely. First-line endoscopic treatments are botulinum toxin (Botox) injection and esophageal balloon dilatation.[18] Endoscopic pneumatic balloon dilatation temporarily relieves dysphagia in up to 70% of cases, and is still widely performed because of its relative noninvasiveness. However, it is associated with a potential risk of esophageal perforation (2.5%) and frequent recurrences, The cumulative 5-year remission rate of pneumatic dilatation for achalasia is reported to be between 50% and 70%. If these interventions are ineffective, surgical myotomy is generally indicated. Surgical myotomy was originally reported by Heller in 1913, and consisted of 2 longitudinal cuts of approximately 8 cm on the anterior and posterior esophageal wall, which included an approximately 2-cm cut on the dilated part (esophagus) and a short cut over the cardia into the fundus. This approach suggests that complete release of the LES is mandatory to achieve complete relief from achalasia symptoms. Later, bilateral myotomy was modified to single myotomy, but the basic principle remained unchanged. Although surgical myotomy provides the best solution for esophageal achalasia, it still has limitations and failures. In particular, gastroesophageal reflux disease (GERD) may occur in up to 30% of cases following a Heller myotomy; it is generally considered to require an additional antireflux procedure, such as Dor fundoplication.

Laparoscopic myotomy is a less invasive technique that significantly reduces the morbidity of open surgery.[19] However, it still requires several abdominal incisions and also involves dissection of the normal esophageal hiatus, which may cause potential hiatal hernia.

ENDOSCOPIC MYOTOMY

The concept of endoscopic myotomy for the treatment of achalasia was first reported in a case series in 1980.[20] However, the direct-incision method through the mucosal layer that was used in this study was not considered a safe and reliable approach, and has not been followed further. Pasricha and colleagues[21] reported the possibility of endoscopic myotomy through a submucosal tunnel in a porcine model. Sumiyama and colleagues[22] also reported the technical feasibility of submucosal tunneling in a porcine model, while Perretta and colleagues[23] have also reported the safety and effectiveness of endoscopic submucosal esophageal myotomy in a pig model. Based on this experimental background, the authors have refined the techniques for clinical application to enable performance of endoscopic myotomy in humans, namely, POEM.[1,3]

WHAT ARE THE TECHNICAL DIFFERENCES BETWEEN ESD AND POEM?

ESD was first developed by Ono[11] to resect intramucosal cancers endoscopically in a 1-piece nonfragmented specimen. Mucosal lesions (high-grade dysplasia or intramucosal carcinoma) resected in a single piece allow complete histopathologic assessment, including horizontal spread and vertical infiltration of the tumor. In ESD, the mucosal layer is resected together with a major part of the submucosal layer while the muscular layer is absolutely preserved. Muscle layer and serosa (or adventitia) acts as a barrier against leakage of gastrointestinal fluid toward the mediastinum and peritoneal cavity. If the muscular layer is incidentally disrupted, this indicates perforation of the gastrointestinal wall, which doubtless causes mediastinitis or peritonitis. Perforation should be immediately closed with endoscopic clip(s).

In the POEM procedure, the muscle layer is intentionally dissected and divided. As a result, the mediastinum is eventually open to submucosal space. In the POEM procedure the preserved mucosa works as a strong barrier to isolate gastrointestinal lumen from the mediastinum or peritoneum. The advanced endoscopic technology of POEM enables dissection of the muscle layer through a submucosal tunnel, without tearing the covering mucosa. Complete endoscopic myotomy had never taken place in clinical experience before the development of the POEM procedure.

Finally, what is learned from both ESD and POEM is that if either the mucosa or muscle layer is kept intact, neither peritonitis nor mediastinitis may occur, because either the mucosa or the muscle layer acts as a strong barrier (**Fig. 1**).

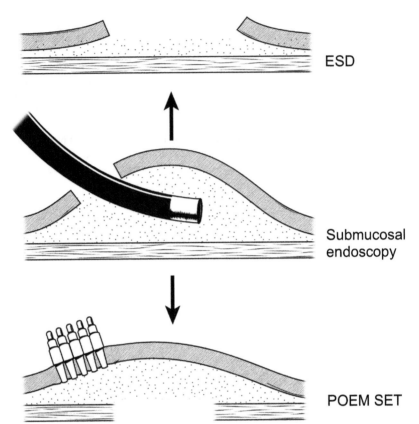

Fig. 1. The mucosa and muscle layers changes during submucosal endoscopy. (*Top*) In ESD (endoscopic submucosal dissection), mucosal layer including mucosal lesion has been removed. Muscle layer is kept intact and it works as a strong barrier. (*Bottom*) In POEM or SET muscle layer eventually has defect but mucosal layer is kept intact. Mucosal layer fascilitates as a tough barrier.

THE POEM PROCEDURE
Equipment Required for POEM

Endoscope and distal attachment
A standard forward-viewing diagnostic gastroscope can be used for the POEM procedure but, if available, a large working-channel (3.2 mm) endoscope with water-jet function is more useful. A transparent distal small tapered cap (ST Hood; Fujifilm, Tokyo, Japan) is preferably attached at the tip of the endoscope. An oblique cap (MH-588; Olympus, Tokyo, Japan) can be used as an alternative. The oblique cap is particularly necessary for clipping the esophageal opening. An overtube is used for stabilization of the endoscope, which effectively avoids mucosal laceration at the mucosal incision site during the POEM procedure. Of course the equipment required for POEM is similar to that needed for ESD.

Carbon dioxide insufflator
CO_2 gas insufflation is essential in achieving a safe POEM procedure. Endoscopic CO_2 insufflation with a controlled gas feed of 1.2 L/min is beneficial for reducing the risk of

both mediastinal emphysema and pneumoperitoneum. The air-supply button should expressly be closed during the procedure, even when the CO_2 insufflator is on. By contrast, ESD can be carried out even under air insufflation, because the muscle layer is kept intact.

Triangle-tip knife

A triangle-tip knife (TT knife) (KD-640 L; Olympus) is used for submucosal tunneling and myotomy. The triangle plate at the tip of the TT knife has 3 angulations, which allow spraying of energy toward a wide circumferential range. Submucosal dissection is effectively carried out without any contact of the TT knife with the tissue.

Electrocautery generator

A high-frequency electrosurgical energy generator (VIO 300D; ERBE Elektromedizin GmbH, Tubingen, Germany, or ESG 400; Olympus) that has a spray coagulation mode with noncontact tissue dissection is effectively used in combination with the TT knife. Spray coagulation mode, effect 2, 50 W, is the best match for TT knife for both submucosal dissection and myotomy. Settings should be individually adjusted during the operation.

Coagulation forceps

Monopolar coagulating forceps (Coagrasper, FD-411QR; Olympus) are used for hemostasis and coagulation of large vessels, when encountered during dissection. The preferred energy setting is soft coagulation 80 W, effect 2.

POEM Procedure

The following technical details of the POEM procedure are consistent with those from original reports.[1,3,24,25]

Step 1: general anesthesia and CO_2 insufflation through the endoscope

POEM is performed under general anesthesia with endotracheal intubation, keeping the patient in the supine position. CO_2 insufflation is mandatory to perform a safe POEM procedure. CO_2 insufflation theoretically avoids pneumomediastinum and air embolization. It is very important to ensure that the air-feeding button on the endoscopy unit is closed during the entire procedure, even when the CO_2 insufflation switch is turned on. If air is insufflated it might cause catastrophic complications. To prevent abdominal compartment syndrome, the upper abdomen is checked periodically during the procedure. When the abdomen is excessively distended, abdominal wall puncture will be performed using an injection needle so as not to allow development of abdominal compartment syndrome.

Step 2: submucosal tunneling

After injection of saline with indigo carmine dye, a 2-cm longitudinal incision is created on the anterior wall. A submucosal tunnel is generally created at anterior wall with one-third circumferential dissection of esophageal lumen.

Myotomy at the 2 o'clock position continuing toward the lesser curve of the stomach potentially avoids damage to the sling collar muscle, which is major component of the angle of His. The angle of His is considered a natural anatomic barrier to postoperative GERD. The estimated length of the submucosal tunnel, although individualized, becomes approximately 16 cm (from 29 to 45 cm from patient's teeth). If patients have abnormal contractions of the upper esophagus, myotomy is extended toward the proximal side. The authors' longest documented myotomy is 25 cm.

Step 3: endoscopic myotomy

Dissection of the circular muscle bundle is usually started at the level of 2 cm distal to the mucosal entry point in the submucosal tunnel, as the standard length of myotomy is more than 10 cm (average 13 cm). A TT knife permits selective dissection of the inner circular muscle layer, which potentially avoids incidental damage to the mediastinal critical organ. In other words, preserving the longitudinal muscle layer is a safety margin of myotomy. All processes can be done under direct endoscopic visual control, and careful dissection is a simple but critical way to maintain safety during the procedure. In initial myotomy, the thickness of the circular muscle cannot be predicted; therefore, it is advisable to begin myotomy by careful step-by-step dissection until the longitudinal muscle layer is identified at the bottom of the myotomy site. Even though the outer longitudinal muscle layer has been preserved, it is thin enough to split just by CO_2 insufflation or a subtle touch of endoscopy. Circular muscle dissection advances from proximal to distal, maintaining the correct dissection plane. The myotomy is extended for a distance of 2 cm toward the stomach. Myotomy at the narrow esophagogastric junction (EGJ) has a higher risk of incidental mucosal damage, although repeated submucosal injection may work as a cushion to potentially avoid it. Smooth passage of the endoscope through the EGJ at the end of myotomy provides immediate confirmation of complete myotomy. At the LES, particular attention should be paid to ensuring that all circular muscle bundles responsible for achalasia are completely cut.

In laparoscopic Heller myotomy, the surrounding structures (phrenoesophageal ligament) of distal esophagus need to be dissected to expose the abdominal esophagus. This dissection causes potential hiatal hernia, resulting in severe postsurgical GERD. To prevent this, a partial antireflux procedure, such as Dor fundoplication, is routinely performed. By contrast, no antireflux procedure is needed after the POEM procedure, because the original hiatal attachments and the acute angle of His are left untouched and the flap-valve mechanism is kept intact.

Another major advantage of POEM is the flexibility of myotomy length. In POEM, myotomy is routinely more than 10 cm, with at least 1 cm cut to the gastric side. In laparoscopic surgery a limited length with a maximum of 10 cm is requisite, because there is limited exposure of the distal esophagus in laparoscopic vision. In cases with vigorous achalasia or diffuse esophageal spasm, long myotomy is recommended. The longest myotomy in the authors' series reached 25 cm with minimal technical difficulty. In the POEM procedure the direction of myotomy can also be set flexibly. In cases of previous surgical failure, posterior myotomy is recommended to avoid access to scar site from previous surgery.

After completion of the myotomy, complete LES relaxation is confirmed by retroflex view of the cardia.

Step 4: closure of mucosal entry

Before closing the mucosal entry, 10 mL saline with 80 mg gentamycin is sprayed into the submucosal tunnel. The stomach should also be emptied of fluid and gas. The mucosal entry site, which is usually 2 to 3 cm long, is closed with 5 to 10 endoscopic clips. The first clip should be placed at the distal end of the longitudinal opening to create a mucosal fold. This fold is used as a guide for placing the next clip. The span between 2 clips is about 3 mm. Successful closure of mucosal entry can be confirmed through endoscopic visualization. Even when mucosal entry is elongated over the myotomy site, tight mucosal closure with clips is necessary to avoid leakage of esophageal contents into the mediastinum.

AN EXTENSION OF POEM: SUBMUCOSAL ENDOSCOPIC TUMOR RESECTION

The substantial clinical success of POEM has encouraged another application of the submucosal tunneling method. Submucosal endoscopic tumor resection is an offshoot of POEM.[4] This technique has also been reported contemporaneously as submucosal tunneling endoscopic resection.[26] Submucosal tumors such as leiomyoma and gastrointestinal stromal tumor can be resected endoscopically through submucosal tunnels. In these procedures, keeping the mucosal layer intact is the key to avoiding mediastinal contamination, but even when mucosal tears occur, tight closure by endoscopic clipping devices secures sealing of the mediastinum from gastrointestinal luminal content. A report of successful full-layer resection of an aberrant pancreas in the esophagus supports this concept.[4]

REFERENCES

1. Inoue H, Minami H, Kobayashi Y, et al. Peroral endoscopic myotomy (POEM) for esophageal achalasia. Endoscopy 2010;42:265–71.
2. Kalloo AN, Singh VK, Jagannath SB, et al. Flexible transgastric peritoneoscopy: a novel approach to diagnostic and therapeutic interventions. Gastrointest Endosc 2004;60:114–7.
3. Inoue H, Minami H, Satodate H, et al. First clinical experience of submucosal endoscopic myotomy for esophageal achalasia with no skin incision. Gastrointest Endosc 2009;69:AB122.
4. Inoue H, Ikeda H, Hosoya T, et al. Submucosal endoscopic tumor resection for subepithelial tumors in the esophagus and cardia. Endoscopy 2012;44:225–30.
5. Dehyle P, Largiader F, Jenny S. A method for endoscopic electroresection of sessile colonic polyps. Endoscopy 1973;5:38–40.
6. Inoue H, Takeshita K, Hori H, et al. Endoscopic mucosal resection with a cap-fitted panendoscope for esophagus, stomach, and colon mucosal lesions. Gastrointest Endosc 1993;39:58–62.
7. Stiegmann CV. Endoscopic ligation: now and the future. Gastrointest Endosc 1993;39:203–5.
8. Chaves DM, Sakai P, Mester M, et al. A new endoscopic technique for the resection of flat polypoid lesions. Gastrointest Endosc 1994;40:224–6.
9. Satodate H, Inoue H, Yoshida T, et al. Circumferential EMR of carcinoma arising in Barrett's esophagus: case report. Gastrointest Endosc 2003;58:288–92.
10. Ell C, May A, Grossner L, et al. Endoscopic mucosal resection of early cancer and high-grade dysplasia in Barrett's esophagus. Gastroenterology 2000;118:670–7.
11. Ono H. Early gastric cancer: diagnosis, pathology, treatment techniques and treatment outcomes. Eur J Gastroenterol Hepatol 2006;18:863–7.
12. Mikaeli J, Islami F, Malekzadeh R. Achalasia: a review of Western and Iranian experiences. World J Gastroenterol 2009;15:5000–9.
13. Gockel HR, Schumacher J, Gockel I, et al. Achalasia: will genetic studies provide insights? Hum Genet 2010;128:353–64.
14. Campos GM, Vittinghoff E, Rabl C, et al. Endoscopic and surgical treatments for achalasia: a systematic review and meta-analysis. Ann Surg 2009;249:45–57.
15. Ahmed A. Achalasia: what is the best treatment? Ann Afr Med 2008;7:141–8.

16. Allescher HD, Storr M, Seige M, et al. Treatment of achalasia: botulinum toxin injection vs pneumatic balloon dilation. A prospective study with long-term follow-Up. Endoscopy 2001;33:1007–17.
17. Carter JT, Nguyen D, Roll GR, et al. Predictors of long-term outcome after laparoscopic esophagomyotomy and Dor fundoplication for achalasia. Arch Surg 2011;146:1024–8.
18. Francis DL, Katzka DA. Achalasia: update on the disease and its treatment. Gastroenterology 2010;139:369–74.
19. Shimi S, Nathanson LK, Cuschieri A. Laparoscopic cardiomyotomy for achalasia. J R Coll Surg Edinb 1991;36:152–4.
20. Ortega JA, Madureri V, Perez I. Endoscopic myotomy in the treatment of achalasia. Gastrointest Endosc 1980;26:8–10.
21. Pasricha PJ, Hawari R, Ahmed I, et al. Submucosal endoscopic esophageal myotomy: a novel experimental approach for the treatment of achalasia. Endoscopy 2007;39:761–4.
22. Sumiyama K, Gostout CJ, Rajan E, et al. Submucosal endoscopy with mucosal flap safety valve. Gastrointest Endosc 2007;65:688–94.
23. Perretta S, Dallemagne B, Donatelli G, et al. Transoral endoscopic esophageal myotomy based on esophageal function testing in a survival porcine model. Gastrointest Endosc 2011;73:111–6.
24. Inoue H, Tianle KM, Ikeda H, et al. Peroral endoscopic myotomy for esophageal achalasia: technique, indication, and outcomes. Thorac Surg Clin 2011;21: 519–25.
25. Eleftheriadis N, Inoue H, Ikeda H, et al. Training in peroral endoscopic myotomy (POEM) for esophageal achalasia. Ther Clin Risk Manag 2012;8:329–42.
26. Xu MD, Lu W, Li QL, et al. Application and evaluation of submucosal tunneling endoscopic resection of gastric submucosal tumors originating from the muscularis propria layer. Zhonghua Wei Chang Wai Ke Za Zhi 2012;15:671–4 [in Chinese].

Investigating Deeper
Muscularis Propria to Natural Orifice Transluminal Endoscopic Surgery

Kazuki Sumiyama, MD, PhD[a],*, Christopher J. Gostout, MD[b],
Hisao Tajiri, MD, PhD[a,c]

KEYWORDS

- Submucosal endoscopy with a mucosal flap safety valve technique
- Intramural endoscopy • Muscularis propria • Enteric nerve system
- Endomicroscopy • Peroral endoscopic myotomy • Submucosal tumor removal
- Submucosal endoscopy with mucosal resection

KEY POINTS

- Submucosal endoscopy with a mucosal flap (SEMF) safety valve technique is a global concept that uses the submucosa as a free working space for endoscopic interventions.
- A purposefully created intramural space provides an endoscopic access route to the deeper layers and into the extraluminal cavities.
- The mucosa overlying the intramural space is protective, reducing contamination during natural orifice transluminal endoscopic surgery (NOTES) procedures and providing a sealant flap to repair the entry point and the submucosal space.
- In addition to NOTES, SEMF has been used to enable endoscopic achalasia myotomy; histologic analysis of the muscularis propria, including neural components; and submucosal tumor removal.

INTRODUCTION

Research into endoscopic tissue excision has focused on pursuing methods to obtain larger specimens.[1] The eventual development of endoscopic submucosal dissection (ESD) enabled radical en bloc removal of a mucosal lesion regardless of size. During efforts to accomplish widespread endoscopic mucosal resection (EMR) in the Mayo

Disclosures: The authors disclosed no financial relationships relevant to this publication.
[a] Department of Endoscopy, The Jikei University School of Medicine, 3-25-8 Nishi Shinbashi, Minato-ku, Tokyo 105-8461, Japan; [b] Developmental Endoscopy Unit, Division of Gastroenterology and Hepatology, Mayo Clinic College of Medicine, 200 First Street Southwest, Rochester, MN 55905, USA; [c] Division of Gastroenterology and Hepatology, Department of Internal Medicine, The Jikei University School of Medicine, 3-25-8 Nishi Shinbashi, Minato-ku, Tokyo 105-8461, Japan
* Corresponding author.
E-mail address: kaz_sum@jikei.ac.jp

Clinic Developmental Endoscopy Unit (DEU), the authors observed that the mucosa could be separated from the underlying submucosa (ie, delamination) with relative ease.[2] The potential value of delamination later resurfaced. Natural orifice transluminal endoscopic surgery (NOTES) established a path for flexible endoscopy beyond the gut wall.[3] During the NOTES experience, the authors recognized that with delamination of the mucosa from the submucosa, the submucosal layer could be converted into a practical endoscopic working space. Pilot animal studies demonstrated that a purposefully created free space within the submucosa would provide off-set tunneled access to the deeper layers as well as a safer and cleaner portal into the extraluminal cavities for NOTES procedures compared with direct full-thickness viscerotomy (**Fig. 1**).[4–8] Conversely, once the submucosa has been opened, the overlying mucosa can be excised more safely from inside the submucosa out into the gut lumen. This inside-out technique could be a safer and easier alternative to the current labor-intensive ESD for en bloc resection of mucosal disease.[9]

Intramural endoscopy has attracted great attention internationally. A variety of promising spin-offs have developed and pioneering clinical studies have already revealed practical advantages of this novel application for gastrointestinal (GI) endoscopy.[10]

SUBMUCOSAL ENDOSCOPY WITH MUCOSAL FLAP SAFETY VALVE TECHNIQUE AND OFF-SET ACCESS TO EXTRALUMINAL SPACES FOR NOTES

Submucosal endoscopy with a mucosal flap (SEMF) safety valve technique was devised as a method to convert the submucosa into a working space for endoscopic intervention and to provide an off-set entry point into the extraluminal space to enable NOTES (see **Fig. 1**).[4,8] The unique feature of this technique is the protective function of the overlying mucosa, which minimizes contamination from luminal contents and provides a sealant flap to the submucosal space after any off-set exit from the gut wall into a body cavity (**Fig. 2**).

The submucosal space, or tunnel, in more limited applications of SEMF, requires a 4 to 5 cm length to provide a safety flap valve. In the authors' experience, a 5 to 10 cm long tunnel is superior; the greater length acts as an added safety measure during NOTES procedures for less risk of extraluminal contamination.[6,7] The SEMF procedure is initiated by creation of a submucosal fluid cushion (SFC) to access the submucosa and initiate the anticipated route of the submucosal tunnel. The SFC is critical for entering the dissection plane and for preventing inadvertent full-thickness injury. Saline works well for quick procedures; however, viscous solutions,

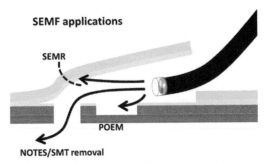

Fig. 1. Submucosal endoscopy with a mucosal flap (SEMF) safety valve technique. NOTES, natural orifice transluminal endoscopic surgery; POEM, peroral endoscopic myotomy; SEMR, submucosal endoscopy with mucosal resection; SMT, submucosal tumor.

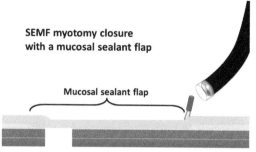

SEMF myotomy closure
with a mucosal sealant flap

Mucosal sealant flap

Fig. 2. SEMF myotomy closure with a mucosal sealant flap. A myotomy created within the SEMF space repaired with an overlaying mucosal flap and endoclip closure of the luminal side mucosal entry point.

such as hyaluronate and hydroxypropyl methylcellulose, remain localized longer, creating a durable SFC and avoiding of supplemental injections. To supplement the SFC and facilitate dissection, a thiol compound, mesna, can be added to the injectate. Mesna chemically softens the submucosa and facilitates dissection by dissolving the disulfide bonds of protein fibers.[11,12] Due to the lack of viscosity, mesna must be used in combination with one of the viscous solutions mentioned above. Following instillation of the SFC, a 5 to 10 mm mucosal incision is made with a needle knife to pass tools through for the actual submucosal dissection. The direction of the mucosal incision is horizontal for a gastric tunnel, to avoid tearing the mucosal incision during the dissection and to ease closure. It is longitudinal for an esophageal tunnel, primarily to facilitate clip closure within the narrow esophageal lumen. Once the early submucosal space is made large enough to accommodate inserting the tip of the endoscope, the dissection is continued with the tip of the scope inside the expanding submucosal tissue space. A transparent cap can aid visualization of the dissection plane. The traditional ESD technique using repetitive electrosurgical dissection can be used to create a tunnel. The tunnel size is ideally restricted to the minimum necessary for endoscopic insertion to preserve the blood supply of the overlying mucosal sealant flap and avoid inadvertent coagulation necrosis of the protective mucosa flap.

In developmental investigations, the authors recognized that the blunt balloon dissection technique provides instant mechanical cleavage of the submucosal tissue plane and facilitates creation of a longitudinal tunnel.[4] Repetitive balloon dissection with a biliary retrieval balloon catheter was originally used with success. A unique cylindrical balloon dissector has been designed for efficient tunnel creation (SuMO, Apollo Endosurgery, Austin, TX) (**Fig. 3**).[13] Initially, the self-advancing hydraulic balloon is stowed within the catheter sheath, unfolding as it advances and distends. The advancing balloon follows the submucosal tissue plane, readily cleaving it without wire guidance. A submucosal tunnel up to 10 cm can be immediately created with a single balloon expansion (**Fig. 4**). The width of the tunnel can be controlled with the variation of the balloon diameter. Although significant bleeding has not been encountered, balloon compression may incidentally provide a hemostatic effect. It has yet to be investigated whether the mechanical balloon dissection technique can completely replace traditional needle knife dissection. Future study should ensure that balloon dissection is effective in the setting of mucosal scaring (without damaging the overlaying mucosa and the muscularis). The submucosal space is readily closed without special skills with simple approximation of the mucosal entry point using endoclips after the decompression of the tunnel

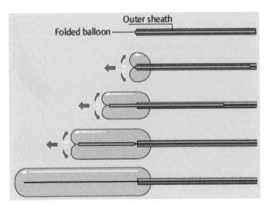

Fig. 3. The balloon tip self-advancing into the submucosal tissue plane by blunt dissection without wire-guidance. (*From* Dobashi A, Sumiyama K, Gostout CJ, et al. Can mechanical balloon dissection be applied to cleave fibrotic submucosal tissues? A pilot study in a porcine model. Endoscopy 2013;45:663; with permission.)

(see **Fig. 2**). Using SEMF as an off-set access for NOTES (gastric) viscerotomy, we were able to directionally perform the submucosal tunneling to direct the endoscope to the gallbladder and perform a cholecystectomy. Although access to the upper abdominal cavity higher than the level of the stomach is inherently restrictive for any transgastric approach because of the mechanical limitations imposed by current flexible endoscopes, the creation of a cephalad submucosal tunnel in retroflexed position overcomes the difficulties with direct transgastric access to the upper abdominal cavity.[6] Kitano and colleagues[14] reported the first clinical experience of anterior transgastric peritoneal access through the cephalad submucosal tunnel created with traditional needle knife dissection. Peritoneoscopy under general anesthesia with laparoscopic monitoring was performed as a part of the preoperative evaluation of patients who have pancreatic cancer.

Combined porcine and cadaver studies revealed that the thoracic cavity from the level of the 4th to the 12th thoracic vertebra is also accessible from the esophagus at the level of the lower esophageal sphincter just above the esophageal hiatus of the diaphragm (distal esophagus).[5,7,15] Key major thoracic organs, including the lung, vertebra, azygos vein, vagus nerve, lymph nodes, and even the heart, can be

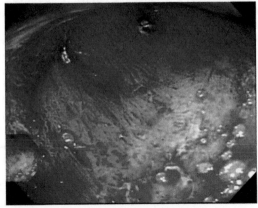

Fig. 4. A free submucosal space mechanically created with the cylindrical balloon dissector.

endoscopically accessed via the transesophageal SEMF approach in porcine models or humans, although technical feasibility has yet to be clinically investigated.

INTRAMURAL ENDOSCOPY FOR DEEPER LAYER VISUALIZATION

Endoscopic optical image resolution has evolved to allow information that is more detailed than imaging of the mucosal surface. Endoscopic ultrasound (EUS) permits monochromatic cross-sectional imaging of the deeper layers, and EUS-guided fine-needle aspiration (EUS-FNA) biopsy enables deeper-lying tissues to be sampled and histologically analyzed. However, the diagnosis of benign diseases, such as functional disorders, is virtually impossible to image with EUS or FNA alone.

The authors used endomicroscopy technologies within the SEMF submucosal space to accomplish in vivo histologic analysis of the deeper layers as a minimally invasive alternative to the ex vivo histology of sampled specimens. To explore the technical feasibility of the endoscopic visualization of intramural structures at the subcellular level, we initially used optical endomicroscopy (Endocytoscopy, Olympus Medical Systems, Tokyo, Japan) in porcine models.[16] This pilot study demonstrated that each spindle-shaped cell body and nucleus of actively contracting smooth muscle cells could be identified in real-time using toluidine blue staining with image resolution equivalent to bench microscopy. Subsequently, confocal laser endomicroscopy (CLE) was used with the intention of visualizing the enteric neural networks.[17] The authors surmised that in vivo confocal imaging could transfer basic bench science into direct, flexible, endoscopic observation of neuromuscular anatomic details and the function of pathognomonic tissues by using specific molecular probes. The authors' animal research proved that the muscularis propria and the enteric mural neural elements could be imaged in vivo, supplemented with neuronal fluorescent stains such as NeuroTrace (Invitrogen, Carlsbad, CA) and cresyl violet (**Fig. 5**). The technical feasibility of CLE imaging of the deeper layers in the human body has now been confirmed clinically.[18] In the inaugural experience, the observation of posttherapeutic ulcerations after endoscopic removal of mucosal lesions was observed with CLE following topical application of acriflavine. The authors believe that this novel in vivo histologic imaging method will provide essential etiologic information and provide solutions that are more reliable for functional GI motility diseases.

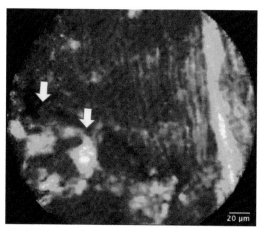

Fig. 5. Confocal endomicroscopy of myenteric ganglion cells in a porcine stomach. Polygonal ganglion cells visualized in the intermuscular tissues (*yellow arrows*).

INTRAMURAL THERAPEUTIC INVENTIONS: ACHALASIA MYOTOMY, MYOMECTOMY FOR SUBMUCOSAL TUMOR REMOVAL, AND SUBMUCOSAL ENDOSCOPY WITH MUCOSAL RESECTION

During our work with SEMF-style NOTES access, we recognized that the muscular layer could be safely sampled from within the submucosal tunnel. We anticipated that this intramural muscular sampling technique might replace the Heller myotomy for the treatment of achalasia.[5] The Apollo group, a multicenter research group established to intensively promote the development of flexible endoscopy and ground-breaking endoscopic interventions such as NOTES, commissioned one of the members with an established career interest in achalasia, Jay Pasricha, to formally design and conduct an animal study to evaluate the technical feasibility of the SEMF myotomy for achalasia.[19] The experiment successfully demonstrated the value of the SEMF technique combined with the selective subtotal incision of the inner circular layer of the lower esophageal sphincter (LES) in the treatment of achalasia by significantly reducing LES pressure in a porcine model. The efficacy and safety of the SEMF-style submucosal subtotal myotomy technique was then clinically confirmed in achalasia patients by Inoue and colleagues[20] at Showa University in Japan. An advantage of this procedure is that a prophylactic antireflux procedure is unnecessary because the endoluminal approach does not disrupt paraesophageal support structures. These play a key role in preventing reflux and they are always dissected in the Heller operation to access the muscularis of the lower esophagus and the gastric cardia. The procedure, now known as peroral endoscopic myotomy (POEM), has become more popular internationally. The Showa University group has already successfully treated hundreds of patients without significant complications or sequelae. The procedure is now universally accepted as a desirable, minimally invasive, therapeutic option for achalasia.[21–28] See the article by Inoue elsewhere in this issue for further discussion of POEM.

When we examined the feasibility of transesophageal thoracic access as described previously, we created a full-thickness muscular layer perforation as a portal site.[5,7] A large muscularis defect greater than 2 cm in size could be sealed securely with a robust and reliable overlying squamous cell mucosal flap. We applied the cap assisted EMR (EMR-C) technique onto the muscularis within the SEMF space in anticipation that the suction and snare myotomy would effectively limit any inadvertent surrounding organ injuries. A subsequent Mayo Clinic DEU study also showed that the EMR-C myotomy provides a sample size with an opportunity to histologically and more comprehensively analyze the myenteric neural network.[13] Full-thickness myotomy, with or without cap initiation, may be technically easier and may strengthen the therapeutic effect in achalasia compared with subtotal myotomy.[29]

Excisions of the muscular layer using SEMF have been modified to accommodate excision of tumors arising from the deeper layers.[30,31] Needle knife dissection is used in this approach to separate the seromuscular plane. Considering the risk for overlaying muscle flap necrosis and stricture in small lumens, tumor size is restricted to less than half of the circumference of the lumen with this technique. At an outpatient endoscopy unit, Lee and colleagues[30] successfully performed the excision of a tumor arising from the muscularis inside the SEMF space using conscious sedation without tracheal intubation.

The overlying mucosa can be removed by simply switching the direction of incision from the muscularis to the opposite way in the gut lumen (see **Fig. 1**) to address en bloc excision of mucosal disease (dysplasia).[9] The submucosal endoscopy with mucosal resection (SEMR) technique may greatly reduce the risk of perforation compared with EMR and ESD. In these traditional techniques, electrocautery is unavoidably directed at the muscularis. Porcine model experiments have already demonstrated the technical safety of SEMR, and traditional ESD is currently being compared with SEMR in animal testing.

SUMMARY

Intramural endoscopic activities illustrate and are reminders of the many interventions to be pursued from within the gut wall. In fact, an array of common GI diseases is attributed to abnormalities within the submucosa and the outermost muscularis propria. The authors believe that intramural procedures will mature and may solve some longstanding issues in gastroenterology.

REFERENCES

1. Sumiyama K, Gostout CJ. Novel techniques and instrumentation for EMR, ESD, and full-thickness endoscopic luminal resection. Gastrointest Endosc Clin N Am 2007;17(3):471–85, v–vi.
2. Rajan E, Gostout CJ, Feitoza AB, et al. Widespread EMR: a new technique for removal of large areas of mucosa. Gastrointest Endosc 2004;60(4):623–7.
3. ASGE, SAGES. ASGE/SAGES Working Group on Natural Orifice Translumenal Endoscopic Surgery White Paper October 2005. Gastrointest Endosc 2006; 63(2):199–203.
4. Sumiyama K, Gostout CJ, Rajan E, et al. Submucosal endoscopy with mucosal flap safety valve. Gastrointest Endosc 2007;65(4):688–94.
5. Sumiyama K, Gostout CJ, Rajan E, et al. Transesophageal mediastinoscopy by submucosal endoscopy with mucosal flap safety valve technique. Gastrointest Endosc 2007;65(4):679–83.
6. Sumiyama K, Gostout CJ, Rajan E, et al. Transgastric cholecystectomy: transgastric accessibility to the gallbladder improved with the SEMF method and a novel multibending therapeutic endoscope. Gastrointest Endosc 2007;65(7): 1028–34.
7. Sumiyama K, Gostout CJ, Rajan E, et al. Pilot study of transesophageal endoscopic epicardial coagulation by submucosal endoscopy with the mucosal flap safety valve technique (with videos). Gastrointest Endosc 2008;67(3):497–501.
8. Sumiyama K, Tajiri H, Gostout CJ. Submucosal endoscopy with mucosal flap safety valve (SEMF) technique: a safe access method into the peritoneal cavity and mediastinum. Minim Invasive Ther Allied Technol 2008;17(6):365–9.
9. Gostout CJ, Knipschield MA. Submucosal endoscopy with mucosal resection: a hybrid endoscopic submucosal dissection in the porcine rectum and distal colon. Gastrointest Endosc 2012;76(4):829–34.
10. Sumiyama K, Gostout CJ. Clinical applications of submucosal endoscopy. Curr Opin Gastroenterol 2011;27(5):412–7.
11. Sumiyama K, Gostout CJ, Rajan E, et al. Chemically assisted endoscopic mechanical submucosal dissection by using mesna. Gastrointest Endosc 2008; 67(3):534–8.
12. Sumiyama K, Tajiri H, Gostout CJ, et al. Chemically assisted submucosal injection facilitates endoscopic submucosal dissection of gastric neoplasms. Endoscopy 2010;42(8):627–32.
13. Rajan E, Gostout CJ, Aimore Bonin E, et al. Endoscopic full-thickness biopsy of the gastric wall with defect closure by using an endoscopic suturing device: survival porcine study. Gastrointest Endosc 2012;76(5):1014–9.

14. Kitano S, Yasuda K, Shibata K, et al. Natural orifice translumenal endoscopic surgery for preoperative staging in a pancreatic cancer patient. Dig Endosc 2008; 20:198–202.
15. Swanstrom LL, Dunst CM, Spaun GO. Future applications of flexible endoscopy in esophageal surgery. J Gastrointest Surg 2010;14(Suppl 1):S127–32.
16. Sumiyama K, Tajiri H, Kato F, et al. Pilot study for in vivo cellular imaging of the muscularis propria and ex vivo molecular imaging of myenteric neurons (with video). Gastrointest Endosc 2009;69(6):1129–34.
17. Ohya TR, Sumiyama K, Takahashi-Fujigasaki J, et al. In vivo histologic imaging of the muscularis propria and myenteric neurons with probe-based confocal laser endomicroscopy in porcine models (with videos). Gastrointest Endosc 2012; 75(2):405–10.
18. Sumiyama K, Kiesslich R, Ohya TR, et al. In vivo imaging of enteric neuronal networks in humans using confocal laser endomicroscopy. Gastroenterology 2012; 143(5):1152–3.
19. Pasricha PJ, Hawari R, Ahmed I, et al. Submucosal endoscopic esophageal myotomy: a novel experimental approach for the treatment of achalasia. Endoscopy 2007;39(9):761–4.
20. Inoue H, Minami H, Kobayashi Y, et al. Peroral endoscopic myotomy (POEM) for esophageal achalasia. Endoscopy 2010;42(4):265–71.
21. Swanstrom LL, Rieder E, Dunst CM. A stepwise approach and early clinical experience in peroral endoscopic myotomy for the treatment of achalasia and esophageal motility disorders. J Am Coll Surg 2011;213(6):751–6.
22. Perretta S, Dallemagne B, Marescaux J. STEPS to POEM: introduction of a new technique at the IRCAD. Surg Innovat 2012;19(3):216–20.
23. Ponsky JL, Marks JM, Pauli EM. How i do it: per-oral endoscopic myotomy (POEM). J Gastrointest Surg 2012;16(6):1251–5.
24. Costamagna G, Marchese M, Familiari P, et al. Peroral endoscopic myotomy (POEM) for oesophageal achalasia: preliminary results in humans. Dig Liver Dis 2012;44(10):827–32.
25. von Renteln D, Inoue H, Minami H, et al. Peroral endoscopic myotomy for the treatment of achalasia: a prospective single center study. Am J Gastroenterol 2012;107(3):411–7.
26. Swanstrom LL, Kurian A, Dunst CM, et al. Long-term outcomes of an endoscopic myotomy for achalasia: the POEM procedure. Ann Surg 2012;256(4):659–67.
27. Chiu PW, Wu JC, Teoh AY, et al. Peroral endoscopic myotomy for treatment of achalasia: from bench to bedside (with video). Gastrointest Endosc 2013;77(1): 29–38.
28. Hungness ES, Teitelbaum EN, Santos BF, et al. Comparison of perioperative outcomes between peroral esophageal myotomy (POEM) and laparoscopic Heller myotomy. J Gastrointest Surg 2013;17(2):228–35.
29. Bonin EA, Moran E, Bingener J, et al. A comparative study of endoscopic full-thickness and partial-thickness myotomy using submucosal endoscopy with mucosal safety flap (SEMF) technique. Surg Endosc 2012;26(6):1751–8.
30. Lee CK, Lee SH, Chung IK, et al. Endoscopic full-thickness resection of a gastric subepithelial tumor by using the submucosal tunnel technique with the patient under conscious sedation (with video). Gastrointest Endosc 2012;75(2):457–9.
31. Inoue H, Ikeda H, Hosoya T, et al. Submucosal endoscopic tumor resection for subepithelial tumors in the esophagus and cardia. Endoscopy 2012;44(3): 225–30.

Regenerative Medicine
Tissue-Engineered Cell Sheet for the Prevention of Post–Esophageal ESD Stricture

Takeshi Ohki, MD, PhD[a,b,*], Masayuki Yamato, PhD[b],
Teruo Okano, PhD[b], Masakazu Yamamoto, MD, PhD[a]

KEYWORDS

- Regenerative medicine • Cell sheet technology • Endoscopic submucosal dissection
- Esophageal stricture • Oral mucosal epithelial cell sheet

KEY POINTS

- Research on the use of regenerative medicine in the gastrointestinal field is gaining momentum around the world.
- In this first-ever clinical study of its type in the gastrointestinal field, a new treatment was developed that involved the transfer of tissue-engineered oral mucosal epithelial cell sheets to post–endoscopic submucosal dissection ulcerations.
- This new treatment showed promising results, indicating that it can potentially prevent post–endoscopic submucosal dissection esophageal stricture.

 Video of the cell sheet transplantation technique accompanies this article

INTRODUCTION

Induced pluripotent stem (iPS) cells, which led to the 2012 Nobel Prize in Physiology or Medicine for Dr Shinya Yamanaka, have captured the world's attention and directed an unprecedented focus on regenerative medicine.[1–3] The potential of iPS cells to

Conflict of Interest: The authors declare no conflicts of interest.
This study was supported by The High-Tech Research Center Program, Formation of Innovation Center for Fusion of Advanced Technologies in the Special Coordination Funds for Promoting Science and Technology "Cell Sheet Tissue Engineering Center (CSTEC)" and the Global COE program, the Multidisciplinary Education and Research Center for Regenerative Medicine (MERCREM), from the Ministry of Education, Culture, Sports, Science and Technology (MEXT), Japan.
[a] Department of Surgery, Institute of Gastroenterology, Tokyo Women's Medical University, 8-1 Kawada-cho, Shinjuku-ku, Tokyo 162-8666, Japan; [b] Institute of Advanced Biomedical Engineering and Science, Tokyo Women's Medical University (TWIns), 8-1 Kawada-cho, Shinjuku-ku, Tokyo 162-8666, Japan
* Corresponding author. Department of Surgery, Institute of Gastroenterology, Tokyo Women's Medical University, 8-1 Kawada-cho, Shinjuku-ku, Tokyo 162-8666, Japan.
E-mail address: ohki@ige.twmu.ac.jp

Gastrointest Endoscopy Clin N Am 24 (2014) 273–281
http://dx.doi.org/10.1016/j.giec.2013.11.003
1052-5157/14/$ – see front matter © 2014 Elsevier Inc. All rights reserved.

aid in the development of new treatments for various diseases is very exciting, and researchers are only beginning to discover their potential benefits for humans. iPS cells are more effective if they are interconnected with tissues; however, new technologies are needed to create and transplant these tissues. In the field of regenerative medicine, clinical research involving cell sheet technology has already been conducted.[4–6] This study introduces a new connection between endoscopy and regenerative medicine in gastroenterology through specifically addressing how cell sheet technology can be a viable method of tissue creation and transplantation.

POST–ENDOSCOPIC SUBMUCOSAL DISSECTION ESOPHAGEAL STRICTURE

Esophageal endoscopic submucosal dissection (ESD) has recently become a standard endoscopic treatment technique,[7–11] similar to gastric ESD.[12–14] However, after a large esophageal ESD, esophageal stricture often arises because of large artificial ulceration.[15,16] A severe esophageal stricture occurring after ESD is difficult to treat and can require frequent endoscopic balloon dilations.[17] Limitations regarding not only the depth but also the size of the tumor exist in the guidelines of the Japan Esophageal Society on the application of endoscopic resection. Ono and colleagues[18] reported that 90% of patients with lesions more than three-fourths the circumference of the esophagus experienced stricture after ESD. Recently, reports on steroid use for esophageal stricture have been increasing[19–22]; however, this has been accompanied by many problems, such as delayed wound healing, immune suppression, optical damage, psychiatric disturbances, diabetes, peptic ulcerations, osteoporosis, and susceptibility to tuberculosis infection. The authors developed a procedure involving the endoscopic transplantation of cultured autologous oral mucosal epithelial cell sheets to an ulcer after endoscopic resection in a canine model to assess the degree to which it could prevent post-ESD esophageal stricture.[23,24]

REGENERATIVE MEDICINE IN ENDOSCOPY

The number of reports on regenerative medicine in endoscopy and gastroenterology is increasing.[25] Isolated oral mucosal epithelial cells have been injected into the submucosal tissue after esophageal endoscopic mucosal resection (EMR) in a porcine model.[26] Epithelialization of the ulceration was confirmed 2 weeks after the injection of epithelial cells. Autologous adipose tissue–derived stromal cells that were not cultured were endoscopically injected into submucosal tissue after esophageal EMR in a canine model.[27] The epithelialization of ulcerations was determined to be promoted by autologous adipose tissue–derived stromal cells. The tubular scaffold of the decellularized porcine urinary bladder has been shown to attach, as if through biologic glue, to the surface of a circumferential ulceration after multiple EMRs in a canine model.[28] Furthermore, the subsequent placement of a scaffold made of a decellularized xenogeneic extracellular matrix (ECM) promoted a constructive remodeling response and minimized stricture.[29]

CELL SHEET TECHNOLOGY

A temperature-responsive polymer [poly(N-isopropylacrylamide)] covalently bound to the surface of a temperature-responsive culture dish has been used as a cell sheet.[30] The culture dish was coated with the temperature-responsive polymer that had a hydrophobic surface at 37°C (normal culture conditions), allowing cells to attach to the surface of the dish (**Fig. 1A**). When the temperature was reduced to 32°C, the surface of the temperature-responsive culture dish became hydrophilic, and the cells

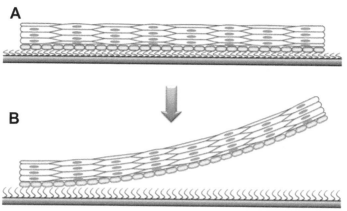

Fig. 1. (*A*) Confluent epithelial cells on temperature-responsive culture surfaces at 36°C. (*B*) Harvesting of the epithelial cell sheets as consecutive cells after a temperature decrease to 20°C.

were released from the dish. The adhesion molecules that maintain contact between cells can be destroyed through the conventional method of freeing cells from the dish using proteases. In contrast, all of the cells can be removed as a continuous sheet along with the extracellular matrix deposited at the base of the culture dish using a temperature-responsive dish (see **Fig. 1**B). Because adhesion molecules are retained on the surface of the cells,[31] the cell sheet can be transplanted onto various tissues without sutures by attaching it for a short period.[4,5] The number of cells used in single-cell injections is low, whereas the scaffolding technique has no cell content, relying on confluent cells for healing to occur. Cell sheets contain high cell density and can also be used to transplant stem cells.

TREATMENT USING AUTOLOGOUS ORAL MUCOSAL EPITHELIAL CELL SHEETS FOR THE PREVENTION OF STRICTURE

The authors developed a regenerative medical treatment using tissue-engineered epithelial cell sheets.[23,32] Epithelial cells isolated from the patient's own oral mucosa[33] were seeded[c] onto temperature-responsive culture inserts[34–36] and cultured[d] for 16 days at 36°C (**Fig. 2**[1–2]). Then, the autologous cell sheets (**Figs. 3** and **4**) were

---

[c] Oral mucosal epithelial cells were collected by remove of epithelial layers after treatment with 1000 U/ml dispase (Godo Shusei, Tokyo, Japan) at 37°C for 2 hours. Epithelial layers were carefully removed from the substantia propria by surgical forceps and treated with 0.25% trypsin/0.1% ethylenediamine tetraacetic acid (EDTA) (GIBCO-Invitrogen, Carlsbad, CA, USA) for 20 minutes at 37°C. Isolated epithelial cells were suspended in a keratinocyte culture medium (KCM) composed of a basal mixture of 3 parts Dulbecco's modified Eagle's medium (DMEM) and 1 part nutrient mixture F-12 Ham (Sigma), and supplemented with 2 nmol/L triiodothyronine (Wako Pure Chemicals, Osaka, Japan), 5 µg/mL insulin (Eli Lilly, Indianapolis, IN, USA), 10 ng/mL epidermal growth factor (Higeta Shoyu, Chiba, Japan), 0.4 µg/mL hydrocortisone (Kowa Pharmaceutical, Tokyo, Japan), 1 nM cholera toxin (List Biological Laboratories, Campbell, CA), 0.25 µg/mL amphotericin B (Bristol-Myers Squibb, New York, NY, USA), 40 µg/mL gentamicin (Schering-Plough, Kenilworth, NJ, USA), and 5% autologous human serum.

[d] Suspended epithelial cells were seeded onto temperature-responsive polymer (N-isopropylacrylamide) grafted cell culture inserts (UpCell Insert; CellSeed, Tokyo, Japan) were prepared with the use of commercial cell culture inserts (Falcon; Becton Dickinson, Franklin Lakes, NJ, USA) at a density of 4 to 8×10^4 cells/cm^2, and cultured for 16 days at 37°C in a humidified atmosphere containing 5% CO_2.

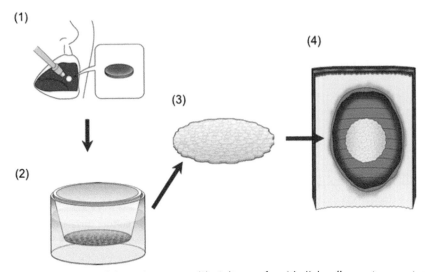

Fig. 2. (1) Biopsies of buccal mucosa. (2) Culture of epithelial cells on temperature-responsive culture inserts for 16 days. (3) Autologous oral mucosal epithelial cell sheets harvested by the reduction in temperature. (4) Endoscopic transplantation of cell sheets immediately after esophageal ESD.

then transplanted with endoscopic forceps onto the bed of the esophageal ulcer after ESD (see **Fig. 2**[3–4]; **Fig. 5**A).[37] The authors reported 9 cases that underwent oral mucosal epithelial cell sheet transplantation.[38] Cell sheet transplantation effectively prevented post-ESD esophageal stricture.

PREPARATION FOR TRANSPLANTATION

The authors used 2 incubators (36°C and 20°C) in an endoscopic room to prepare the cell sheets for transplantation. The cell sheets were carried in a container from a cell

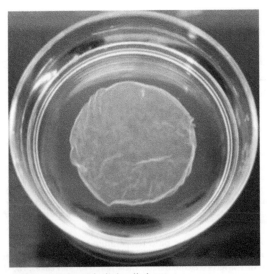

Fig. 3. Autologous oral mucosal epithelial cell sheet.

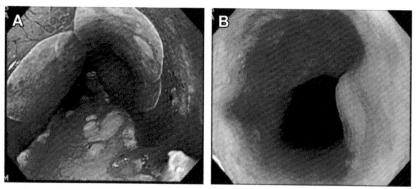

Fig. 4. (*A*) Endoscopic view immediately after endoscopic transplantation of cell sheets. (*B*) Endoscopic view 5 weeks after transplantation.

processing center[39] to the 36°C incubator (see **Fig. 5A**). During ESD, the cell culture team staff carried the sheets to another incubator (20°C) and harvested the cell sheets in a neighboring room. A support membrane was placed on the cell sheet after the culture medium was removed (see **Fig. 5B–C**). The cell sheet was attached to a support membrane, polyvinylidene difluoride (Immobilon-P, Durapore, Millipore, Billerica, MA), in preparation for endoscopic transplantation (see **Fig. 5D**).

TRANSPLANTATION TECHNIQUE

An esophageal EMR tube (Create Medic Co., Ltd, Yokohama, Japan)[40] was inserted into the esophagus before cell sheet transplantation (Video 1). The support membrane

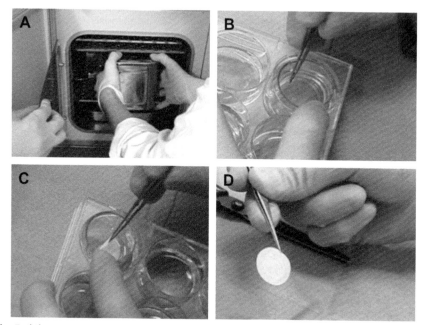

Fig. 5. (*A*) Removing the cell sheet from an incubator in the endoscopic room. (*B*) Trimming confluent epithelial cells at the edge of the cell sheet. (*C*) Attaching the cell sheets to support membranes. (*D*) Grasping the support membrane for endoscopic transplantation.

with the attached autologous oral mucosal epithelial cell sheet was grasped with endoscopic forceps and carefully maneuvered to the ulcer site through the EMR tube. Cell sheets were then placed directly onto the ulcer sites. The cell sheets stably adhered to the ulcer wound beds after at least 10 minutes. The support membrane was not removed, and this procedure was repeated with several transplanted cell sheets to cover the ulcer.

FUTURE DIRECTIONS
Epidermal Epithelial Cell Sheet

Although there are size limitations with oral mucosal cell sheets, epidermal epithelial cell sheets can vary greatly in size because skin extends over a far greater area. Kanai and colleagues[41] reported the effectiveness of epidermal epithelial cell sheets in a swine model, in which stricture was successfully prevented. Another advantage of epidermal epithelial cells is that they are much easier to extract than oral mucosal cell sheets.

Allogeneic Cell Sheet

In the future, allogeneic epithelial cells from a skin bank and artificial skin grafts (AlloDerm [LifeCell Corporation, Branchburg, NJ, USA]) may be used in cell sheet treatments.[42,43] These are particularly advantageous because the removal of oral mucosal tissue is not necessary and they are affordable. Furthermore, the recovery time is much faster because the allogeneic cell sheets promote natural healing.

Development of a Device for Endoscopic Transplantation

Transferring one cell sheet currently takes 10 minutes. Thus, transferring 6 cell sheets takes approximately 1 hour. The authors would like to reduce transplantation time using technology that can transfer many cell sheets simultaneously. If this technology is developed successfully, they believe that cell sheet treatments will be widely used in the gastroenterologic field in the near future.

SUPPLEMENTARY DATA

Video related to this article can be found online at http://dx.doi.org/10.1016/j.giec.2013.11.003.

REFERENCES

1. Takahashi K, Yamanaka S. Induction of pluripotent stem cells from mouse embryonic and adult fibroblast cultures by defined factors. Cell 2006;126:663–76.
2. Takahashi K, Tanabe K, Ohnuki M, et al. Induction of pluripotent stem cells from adult human fibroblasts by defined factors. Cell 2007;131:861–72.
3. Aoi T, Yae K, Nakagawa M, et al. Generation of pluripotent stem cells from adult mouse liver and stomach cells. Science 2008;321:699–702.
4. Yang J, Yamato M, Nishida K, et al. Cell delivery in regenerative medicine: the cell sheet engineering approach. J Control Release 2006;116:193–203.
5. Yang J, Yamato M, Shimizu T, et al. Reconstruction of functional tissues with cell sheet engineering. Biomaterials 2007;28:5033–43.
6. Nishida K, Yamato M, Hayashida Y, et al. Corneal reconstruction with tissue-engineered cell sheets composed of autologous oral mucosal epithelium. N Engl J Med 2004;351:1187–96.

7. Oyama T, Tomori A, Hotta K, et al. Endoscopic submucosal dissection of early esophageal cancer. Clin Gastroenterol Hepatol 2005;3:S67–70.
8. Fujishiro M, Yahagi N, Kakushima N, et al. Endoscopic submucosal dissection of esophageal squamous cell neoplasms. Clin Gastroenterol Hepatol 2006;4: 688–94.
9. Fujishiro M, Kodashima S, Goto O, et al. Endoscopic submucosal dissection for esophageal squamous cell neoplasms. Dig Endosc 2009;21:109–15.
10. Yahagi N. Is esophageal endoscopic submucosal dissection an extreme treatment modality, or can it be a standard treatment modality? Gastrointest Endosc 2008;68:1073–5.
11. Ono S, Fujishiro M, Niimi K, et al. Long-term outcomes of endoscopic submucosal dissection for superficial esophageal squamous cell neoplasms. Gastrointest Endosc 2009;70:860–6.
12. Gotoda T, Kondo H, Ono H, et al. A new endoscopic mucosal resection procedure using an insulation-tipped electrosurgical knife for rectal flat lesions: report of two cases. Gastrointest Endosc 1999;50:560–3.
13. Ono H, Kondo H, Gotoda T, et al. Endoscopic mucosal resection for treatment of early gastric cancer. Gut 2001;48:225–9.
14. Isomoto H, Shikuwa S, Yamaguchi N, et al. Endoscopic submucosal dissection for early gastric cancer: a large-scale feasibility study. Gut 2009;58:331–6.
15. Fujishiro M, Kodashima S, Goto O, et al. Technical feasibility of endoscopic submucosal dissection of gastrointestinal epithelial neoplasms with a splash-needle. Surg Laparosc Endosc Percutan Tech 2008;18:592–7.
16. Takahashi H, Arimura Y, Okahara S, et al. Risk of perforation during dilation for esophageal strictures after endoscopic resection in patients with early squamous cell carcinoma. Endoscopy 2010;43:184–9.
17. Isomoto H, Yamaguchi N, Nakayama T, et al. Management of esophageal stricture after complete circular endoscopic submucosal dissection for superficial esophageal squamous cell carcinoma. BMC Gastroenterol 2011;11:46.
18. Ono S, Fujishiro M, Niimi K, et al. Predictors of postoperative stricture after esophageal endoscopic submucosal dissection for superficial squamous cell neoplasms. Endoscopy 2009;41:661–5.
19. Yamaguchi N, Isomoto H, Shikuwa S, et al. Effect of oral prednisolone on esophageal stricture after complete circular endoscopic submucosal dissection for superficial esophageal squamous cell carcinoma: a case report. Digestion 2011;83:291–5.
20. Yamaguchi N, Isomoto H, Nakayama T, et al. Usefulness of oral prednisolone in the treatment of esophageal stricture after endoscopic submucosal dissection for superficial esophageal squamous cell carcinoma. Gastrointest Endosc 2011;73: 1115–21.
21. Ono S, Fujishiro M, Kodashima S, et al. High-dose dexamethasone may prevent esophageal stricture after endoscopic submucosal dissection. Clin J Gastroenterol 2011;3:155–8.
22. Hashimoto S, Kobayashi M, Takeuchi M, et al. The efficacy of endoscopic triamcinolone injection for the prevention of esophageal stricture after endoscopic submucosal dissection. Gastrointest Endosc 2011;74(6):1389–93.
23. Ohki T, Yamato M, Murakami D, et al. Treatment of oesophageal ulcerations using endoscopic transplantation of tissue-engineered autologous oral mucosal epithelial cell sheets in a canine model. Gut 2006;55:1704–10.
24. New technique improves ulcer healing after esophageal ESD. Nat Clin Pract Gastroenterol Hepatol 2007;4:122.

25. Peterson J, Pasricha PJ. Regenerative medicine and the gut. Gastroenterology 2011;141:1162–6, 1166.e1–2.
26. Sakurai T, Miyazaki S, Miyata G, et al. Autologous buccal keratinocyte implantation for the prevention of stenosis after EMR of the esophagus. Gastrointest Endosc 2007;66:167–73.
27. Honda M, Hori Y, Nakada A, et al. Use of adipose tissue-derived stromal cells for prevention of esophageal stricture after circumferential EMR in a canine model. Gastrointest Endosc 2011;73:777–84.
28. Nieponice A, McGrath K, Qureshi I, et al. An extracellular matrix scaffold for esophageal stricture prevention after circumferential EMR. Gastrointest Endosc 2009;69:289–96.
29. Badylak SF, Hoppo T, Nieponice A, et al. Esophageal preservation in five male patients after endoscopic inner-layer circumferential resection in the setting of superficial cancer: a regenerative medicine approach with a biologic scaffold. Tissue Eng Part A 2011;17:1643–50.
30. Okano T, Yamada N, Sakai H, et al. A novel recovery system for cultured cells using plasma-treated polystyrene dishes grafted with poly(N-isopropylacrylamide). J Biomed Mater Res 1993;27:1243–51.
31. Kushida A, Yamato M, Konno C, et al. Decrease in culture temperature releases monolayer endothelial cell sheets together with deposited fibronectin matrix from temperature-responsive culture surfaces. J Biomed Mater Res 1999;45:355–62.
32. Takagi R, Yamato M, Kanai N, et al. Cell sheet technology for regeneration of esophageal mucosa. World J Gastroenterol 2012;18:5145–50.
33. Sasaki R, Yamato M, Takagi R, et al. Punch and spindle-shaped biopsies for collecting oral mucosal tissue for the fabrication of transplantable autologous epithelial cell sheets. J Biomed Mater Res A 2012;100:2849–54.
34. Murakami D, Yamato M, Nishida K, et al. The effect of micropores in the surface of temperature-responsive culture inserts on the fabrication of transplantable canine oral mucosal epithelial cell sheets. Biomaterials 2006;27:5518–23.
35. Murakami D, Yamato M, Nishida K, et al. Fabrication of transplantable human oral mucosal epithelial cell sheets using temperature-responsive culture inserts without feeder layer cells. J Artif Organs 2006;9:185–91.
36. Takagi R, Yamato M, Murakami D, et al. Preparation of keratinocyte culture medium for the clinical applications of regenerative medicine. J Tissue Eng Regen Med 2010;5:e63–73.
37. Takagi R, Murakami D, Kondo M, et al. Fabrication of human oral mucosal epithelial cell sheets for treatment of esophageal ulceration by endoscopic submucosal dissection. Gastrointest Endosc 2010;72:1253–9.
38. Ohki T, Yamato M, Ota M, et al. Prevention of esophageal stricture after endoscopic submucosal dissection using tissue-engineered cell sheets. Gastroenterology 2012;143:582–8.e1–2.
39. Yamato M, Takagi R, Kondo M, et al. Grand Espoir: robotics in regenerative medicine. J Robot Mechatron 2007;19:500–5.
40. Makuuchi H, Yoshida T, Ell C. Four-step endoscopic esophageal mucosal resection (EEMR) tube method of resection for early esophageal cancer. Endoscopy 2004;36:1013–8.
41. Kanai N, Yamato M, Ohki T, et al. Fabricated autologous epidermal cell sheets for the prevention of esophageal stricture after circumferential ESD in a porcine model. Gastrointest Endosc 2012;76:873–81.

42. Wainwright DJ. Use of an acellular allograft dermal matrix (AlloDerm) in the management of full-thickness burns. Burns 1995;21:243–8.
43. Livesey SA, Herndon DN, Hollyoak MA, et al. Transplanted acellular allograft dermal matrix. Potential as a template for the reconstruction of viable dermis. Transplantation 1995;60:1–9.

ESD Around the World: Asia

Mi-Young Kim, MD, PhD[a], Jun-Hyung Cho, MD[a], Pankaj Jain, MD[b],
Joo Young Cho, MD, PhD[a],*

KEYWORDS

- Early gastric cancer • Endoscopic submucosal dissection • Sentinel node navigation
- Hybrid NOTES

KEY POINTS

- Endoscopic submucosal dissection (ESD) improves the quality of life of patients with early gastric cancer (EGC) and dysplasia by preserving gastric function.
- ESD in the treatment of EGC and dysplasia has become standard treatment in Japan and Korea and is being developed and implemented in many major centers in Asia.
- With a well-designed prospective study, long-term outcomes of expanded criteria for endoscopic resection of EGC are expected to provide reliable indications for endoscopic treatment.
- Ongoing and novel clinical investigations of minimally invasive approaches and close collaboration between Western and Asian countries are expected to establish the best way to treat EGC.

INTRODUCTION

Recent advances in endoscopic imaging, such as magnifying endoscopy, narrow band imaging, and high-definition endoscopy, have enabled the detection of gastric cancer and dysplasia at very early stages. In Asian countries like Korea and Japan, where the burden of gastric cancer is high, endoscopic screening for gastric cancer has been especially recommended and implemented early. As a result, the detection rate of early gastric cancer (EGC) and dysplasia has increased.

EGC is defined as gastric cancer confined to the mucosal (T1a) or submucosal layers (T1b), irrespective of the presence of lymph node metastasis.[1,2] The gold standard for treatment of EGC has been gastrectomy with lymph node dissection, because there is no definitive method to confirm the presence of lymph node

[a] Digestive Disease Center, Soonchunhyang University Hospital, Seoul, Korea; [b] Department of Gastroenterology, Sterling Hospital, Vadodara, India
* Corresponding author. Department of Internal Medicine, Soonchunhyang University Hospital Seoul, Soonchunhyang University College of Medicine, 59 Daesagwan-ro, Yongsan-gu, Seoul 140-743, Korea.
E-mail address: cjy6695@dreamwiz.com

Gastrointest Endoscopy Clin N Am 24 (2014) 283–293
http://dx.doi.org/10.1016/j.giec.2013.11.001
1052-5157/14/$ – see front matter © 2014 Elsevier Inc. All rights reserved.

metastasis other than pathologic examination of the lymph nodes. Although minimally invasive procedures such as laparoscopic function-preserving surgery have been developed, surgery for patients with EGC still results in a compromised quality of life. Endoscopic mucosal resection (EMR) is an alternative to gastrectomy for treatment of EGC, with little to no risk of developing lymph node metastasis for those lesions meeting the standard criteria for the EMR procedure.[3] Moreover, the introduction of endoscopic submucosal dissection (ESD) allows clinicians to meet the challenges of size limitation and evaluation of resection margins that are inherent in EMR.[4]

This article reviews the development, outcomes, investigations, and future directions of ESD for EGC in Asia.

DEVELOPMENT OF ESD

EMR has evolved since it was developed in Japan in the 1980s. In 2001, the Japanese Gastric Cancer Association published the standard criteria for EMR of EGC.[5,6] The indications for EMR are (1) well-differentiated elevated cancers less than 2 cm in diameter, and (2) small (<1 cm) depressed lesions without ulceration. These cancers must also be moderately or well differentiated and confined to the mucosa, and they must have no lymphatic or vascular involvement. Further studies by Gotoda and colleagues[7] suggested a lower-risk category, derived from an analysis of 5265 surgical specimens of patients with EGC who underwent gastrectomy with lymph node dissection. That study permitted the criteria for endoscopic resection to be expanded. The expanded criteria are (1) mucosal cancer without ulceration, irrespective of tumor size; (2) mucosal cancer with ulceration less than or equal to 3 cm in diameter; and (3) minimal submucosal invasive cancer less than or equal to 3 cm in size ($\leq$0.5 mm from the muscularis mucosa).

In the late 1990s, ESD was developed for the complete removal of EGC and gastric dysplasia, regardless of size and location. With this technique, the submucosal layer is dissected with through-the-scope endoscopic knives. ESD is superior to EMR because it allows en bloc resection and precise pathologic staging of large gastric lesions. ESD has become standard treatment in both Japan and Korea for EGCs, and it is being used in many major centers in Asia to achieve en bloc resection of premalignant gastric lesions and EGCs that would otherwise require piecemeal or surgical resection.

In Korea, EMR for EGC was introduced in 1996. Since then, several small-scale studies have been reported. The first large-scale, multicenter, retrospective study was reported in 2007; it stated that circumferential precutting followed by snare resection accounted for more than half of all endoscopic resections of EGC.[8] Of these, ESD was used in 6.6%. Since Park and colleagues[9] initially reported 27 cases of ESD using the insulated-tip knife, use of ESD has increased rapidly in Korea, accompanied by an increase in published data for ESD treatment.

ENDOSCOPIC AND PATHOLOGIC OUTCOMES OF ESD

Results of recent studies from Asia have suggested that ESD achieves a high rate of en bloc resection (89.7%–96.7%) and complete resection (87.9%–94.7%) (**Table 1**). A group of Japanese researchers published their multicenter retrospective study in 2006 to determine the nationwide results of endoscopic resection.[10] After patients with undifferentiated mucosal cancer were excluded, a total of 714 EGCs (EMR, 411; ESD, 303) in 655 consecutive patients from 11 Japanese institutions were included in the study. Most of the lesions (71.6%) were resected en bloc. The rate of en bloc resection with ESD was significantly higher than that for EMR (92.7% vs 56.0%). On histology, resection was curative in 66.3% of the lesions, and the rate of curative resection from ESD was significantly higher than that from EMR (73.6% vs 61.1%). Severe bleeding requiring transfusions occurred in 0.1% of cases with EMR. The frequency of perforation with ESD and EMR was 3.6% and 1.2%, respectively. All complications were managed endoscopically, and there were no procedure-related deaths. The median follow-up period was 3.2 years. The 3-year cumulative residual recurrence-free rate in the ESD group was significantly higher than that in the EMR group (97.6% vs 92.5%; $P = .001$).

In another study, a comparison of EMR and ESD in 1020 patients with EGC who met the expanded criteria (EMR, 825; ESD, 195) found that en bloc resection rates and curative resection rates were significantly higher with ESD (both 92.8%) than with EMR (43.4% and 22.6%, respectively) in cases without ulceration, regardless of tumor size.[11] The average procedure time was significantly longer for ESD than for EMR (84.4 minutes vs 12.6 minutes), regardless of tumor size ($P<.001$), and the frequency of intraoperative bleeding was significantly higher with ESD (22.6%) than with EMR (7.6%). However, the frequency of delayed bleeding did not differ, and the disease was not known to recur in any patient.

Another study of the endoscopic and pathologic outcomes of ESD in relation to lesion size, location, and presence or absence of ulceration revealed that the rate of en bloc resection was 93% and the rate of curative resection was 84%, with a perforation rate of 6.1%.[12] The rate of curative en bloc resection varied significantly depending on the location of the lesion in the stomach (upper vs middle vs lower, 74% vs 77% vs 91%), as well as on the size of the lesion (>20 mm vs ≤20 mm, 59% vs 89%).

Chung and colleagues[13] published a large, multicenter, retrospective study of ESD in Korea in 2009. One thousand EGCs in 952 patients were treated by ESD at ESD study group–related university hospitals between January 2006 and June 2007. The rates of en bloc resection, complete resection, vertical incomplete resection, and piecemeal resection were 95.3%, 87.7%, 1.8%, and 4.1%, respectively. The rates of delayed bleeding and perforation were 15.6% and 1.2%, respectively. The rates of en bloc resection differed significantly in relation to the location of the lesions in the stomach (upper portion vs middle portion vs lower portion, 88.6% vs 95.2% vs 96.0%, respectively; $P = .002$), presence of a scar (no vs yes, 96.0% vs 89.5%, respectively; $P = .002$), and histologic type (low-grade adenoma vs high-grade adenoma vs differentiated EGC vs undifferentiated EGC, 95.8% vs 94.6% vs 96.2% vs 83.8%, respectively; $P = .007$). The results suggest that ESD is an effective and safe therapy in the management of early gastric neoplasm in Korea. Several other studies have also shown better outcomes with ESD than with EMR.[14–16]

In Taiwan, a retrospective, multicenter review of ESD of 70 EGCs found that the en bloc resection rate was 91.4% and the local recurrence rate was 2.8%.[17]

A recent meta-analysis to evaluate the efficacy and safety of ESD and EMR for EGC found considerable advantages for ESD regarding en bloc resection rate, histologically complete resection rate, and local nonrecurrence rate, even for small lesions. However, ESD had a higher complication rate because of a higher rate of perforation.[18] In the meta-analysis, a total of 3548 lesions from 9 retrospective studies were evaluated (ESD, 1495; EMR, 2053). The mean time required for resection was longer for ESD than for EMR (weighted mean difference, 59.4; 95% confidence interval [CI], 16.8–102.0). The en bloc resection rate for ESD was significantly higher than for EMR (odds ratio [OR], 9.69; 95% CI, 7.74–12.13), as was the histologically complete resection rate (OR, 5.66; 95% CI, 2.92–10.96). ESD was also associated with a lower rate of recurrence (OR, 0.10; 95% CI, 0.06–0.18). The perforation rate was higher with

Table 1
Therapeutic outcomes of ESD in Asia

Author/ Publication Year	Study Design	No. (Lesion/ Patient)	Method	En Bloc Resection Rate (%)	Complete Resection Rate (%)	Follow-up (mo/Range)	Complications (%) Bleeding	Complications (%) Perforation	Local Recurrence Rate (%)	3-y Residual/ Recurrence-free Rate (%)	3-y Overall Survival Rate (%)	5-y Overall Survival Rate (%)	5-y Disease-free Survival Rate (%)
Oda et al,[10] 2006	Retrospective	714/655	EMR 411 ESD 303	56.0	61.1	38 (6–60)	0.1	1.2	7.5	92.5	99.2	NA	NA
Oka et al,[11] 2006	Retrospective	1020/896	EMR 825 ESD 195	43.4	24.6	83.2	3.9	0.5	3.5	NA	NA	NA	NA
Imagawa et al,[12] 2006	Retrospective	196/185	ESD	93.0	84.0	17.6 (1.3–45.7)	—	6.1	0	NA	NA	NA	NA
Jung et al,[14] 2012	Retrospective	1327/NA	EMR-P 775 ESD 552	NA	91.0 95.1	NA	6.3 7.6	0.8 2.7	NA	NA	NA	NA	NA
Chung et al,[13] 2009	Retrospective	1000/952	ESD	95.3	87.7	NA	15.6	1.2	NA	NA	NA	NA	NA
Jang et al,[15] 2009	Retrospective	402/402 (198 EGC)	ESD	89.7	87.9	30 (9–49)	7.4	2.9	5.1	94.9	NA	NA	NA

Study	Design (treated/followed)	Method			Mean follow-up, mo							
Min et al,[16] 2009	Retrospective 346/243	EMR-P 103	77.77	75.7	29 (4–44)	3.9	1.9	0	NA	NA	NA	NA
Chang et al,[17] 2009	Retrospective 70/70	ESD	91.4	92.8	NA	5.7	4.3	2.8	NA	NA	NA	NA
Isomoto et al,[4] 2009	Retrospective 589/551	ESD	94.9	94.7	30 (6–89)	1.8	4.5	0	NA	>97.2	97.1	100
Goto et al,[19] 2009	Retrospective 276/231	ESD	96.7	91.7	36 (2–93)	5.1	4.0	0.9	99.1	96.2	96.2	100
Nakamoto et al,[20] 2009	Retrospective 202/177	EMR 80 ESD 122	53.8	37.5	54 (12–89)	—	—	17.5	82.5[a]	100	100	100
Choi et al,[21] 2011	Retrospective 1058/1058	EMR 215 Operation 843	—	71.2	81 (56–94)	—	—	—	98.8[a]	—	93.6	—
Ahn et al,[22] 2011	Retrospective 1370/1244	Absolute Ix / Expanded Ix	—	—	32 (22–48)	—	—	0.9 1.1	—	—	95.8–95.3 96.8	—
		EMR 355 / EMR 182	72.4 65.9	94.4 83.0		1.4 1.6	0.3 1.6	1.5 1.6				
		ESD 497 / ESD 336	96.8 95.5	97.8 91.1		0.8 2.1	1.2 2.4	0.5 0.8				

Abbreviations: EMR-P, precutting followed by snare resection; Ix, indication; NA, not applicable.

[a] Overall 5-year recurrence-free rate.

ESD (OR, 4.67; 95% CI, 2.77–7.87), but the bleeding incidence was similar between the two procedures.

To show the efficacy and safety of ESD, all of the results mentioned earlier should be confirmed by well-designed, randomized, controlled trials from more countries, with larger samples and long-term follow-up periods.

ONCOLOGIC OUTCOMES OF ESD

Expanding the indications for ESD has remained controversial because the long-term outcomes of these expanded criteria have not been validated (see **Table 1**). The first long-term follow-up results of ESD, for 589 EGCs that met the expanded criteria, were reported in 2009[4]; en bloc resection and curative resection rates were 94.9% and 94.7%, respectively. Hence, en bloc resection achieved curative resection consistently. Patients with noncurative resections developed local recurrence more frequently. The 5-year overall and disease-free survival rates were 97.1% and 100%, respectively.[4]

Another retrospective study evaluated the long-term outcomes of ESD in 276 node-negative EGCs that met the expanded criteria, with exclusion of undifferentiated types of mucosal cancer; the en bloc and complete resection rates were 96.7% and 91.7%, respectively.[19] During a median follow-up of 3 years, there were 2 local recurrences (0.9%). The 5-year overall survival rate was 96.2% and the disease-specific survival rate was 100%.

In a comparative study of EMR and ESD for 202 EGCs (EMR, 80; ESD, 122), the overall en bloc and complete resection rates were lower in patients undergoing EMR than in those undergoing ESD (en bloc, 53.8% vs 94.3%; complete, 37.5% vs 92.6%, respectively).[20] The overall 5-year recurrence-free rate was lower in the EMR group than in the ESD group (82.5% vs 100%). However, for small lesions (<5 mm), outcomes for EMR and ESD were similar.

A propensity score matching analysis to compare the long-term outcomes after EMR with outcomes after surgery was published in 2011.[21] In the matched cohort, there were no significant differences between the groups in the risk of death (hazard ratio [HR] for the EMR group, 1.39; 95% CI, 0.87–2.23) or recurrence (HR, 1.18; 95% CI, 0.22–6.35). Although patients who underwent EMR had a higher risk of metachronous gastric cancers (HR, 6.72; 95% CI, 2.00–22.58), all recurrent or metachronous cancers after EMR were successfully retreated without affecting overall survival. The EMR group had a significantly shorter hospital stay (median 8 days, interquartile range [IQR] 6–11 days; vs 15 days, IQR 12–19 days; $P<.001$) and lower cost of care ($2049, IQR $1586–2425; vs $4042, IQR $3458–4959; $P<.001$).

Around the same time, endoscopic and oncologic outcomes after EMR and ESD for EGC using absolute or expanded indications in a Korean study were published.[22] Although the complete resection rate was higher (95.9% vs 88.4%; $P<.001$) and the complication rate was lower (6.8% vs 9.8%; $P = .054$) in the absolute-indication group than in the expanded-indication group, there was no between-group difference in the local recurrence rate (0.9% vs 1.1%; $P = .783$) at a median follow-up period of 32 months (IQR, 22–48 months). In the expanded-indication group, ESD resulted in a significantly higher complete resection rate than did EMR (83.0% vs 91.1%; $P = .006$).

ONGOING ISSUES AND FORECAST OF ESD
Management of Noncurative ESD and ESD with High-risk Factors of Recurrence

Current research is focusing on whether patients with incomplete resection after EMR and ESD, confirmed histologically, can be managed with laparoscopic gastrectomy, or even laparoscopic lymph node dissection, without gastrectomy when margins are negative.

In Japan, 45 patients with incomplete EMR for EGC treated surgically were analyzed to elicit the risk of residual cancer and lymph node metastasis.[23] Among them, 21 patients had mucosal cancer and lateral cut-end–positive status with no lymph node metastasis. Eighteen patients had residual cancer, with the lesions in most patients being limited to the mucosal layer. The patients with mucosal cancer with lateral cut-end–positive margins with no nodal metastases were advised to have either close follow-up or additional endoscopic treatment.

In a Korean study, patients with mucosal cancers larger than 3 cm or a submucosal cancer regardless of size or margin involvement were analyzed for residual cancer and lymph node metastasis.[24] Neither residual cancer nor lymph node metastasis was found when less than 500-μm submucosal invasion without margin involvement in endoscopically resected specimens was present. In a study to evaluate predictive factors for lymph node metastasis in EGC with submucosal invasion, lymphatic involvement and tumor size were independent risk factors in 28 patients who underwent curative gastrectomy because of noncurative endoscopic resection for EGC.[25] The rate of residual cancer in the positive lateral margin group (25.0%) was significantly lower than that in the positive vertical margin group (33.3%) or in the positive lateral and vertical margin group (66.7%).[26] Based on the results of these studies, endoscopic resection may be feasible for highly selective submucosal cancers with no lymphatic involvement or minimal submucosal invasion ($\leq$500 μm) and the tumor size is less than 1 cm. Gastrectomy is recommended for patients with positive vertical margins, submucosal involvement having high-risk features, or lymphovascular invasion.

Another area of investigation is laparoscopic lymph node dissection without gastrectomy in patients treated with ESD whose lesions have negative margins but who are considered to be at high risk for lymph node metastasis based on the presence of other criteria (submucosal invasion, lymphovascular invasion, or undifferentiated adenocarcinoma). In a small case series, the area for lymph node dissection was determined by the location of the tumor and/or the lymphatic drainage of the stomach visualized with standard laparoscopy or infrared-ray electronic laparoscopy after submucosal injection of indocyanine green around post-ESD scars. A retrospective study of 21 patients showed that 2 patients (10%) had lymph node metastases confirmed after lymph node dissection without gastrectomy, and none had local or distant recurrence at a median follow-up of 61 months.[27] Thus, this approach may be acceptable for carefully selected patients, but prospective comparison studies are needed to validate this possibility.

Poorly Differentiated and Undifferentiated Adenocarcinomas

In the past, patients with poorly differentiated adenocarcinomas were not considered candidates for endoscopic resection. Therefore, endoscopic management in this circumstance is controversial and has not been evaluated in well-designed, controlled, prospective studies. However, small studies have shown success with ESD for lesions smaller than 20 mm with no lymphovascular invasion.[28,29] Another study, from Korea, showed that poorly differentiated EGC confined to the mucosa or with minimal submucosal infiltration ($\leq$500 μm) could be considered for curative EMR because the risk of lymph node metastasis was low.[30] Moreover, a study by Park and colleagues[31] showed that EGC with signet ring cell histology can be treated by EMR if the cancer is smaller than 25 mm, limited to the submucosal layer ($\leq$1000 μm), and does not involve lymphatic-vascular structures. However, for larger lesions that have submucosal invasion and/or ulceration, curative resection with ESD is less likely to be possible, and traditional surgery or salvage gastrectomy with lymph node dissection is recommended.[32]

ESD with Sentinel Node Navigation

As the indications for endoscopic resection increase, the issue of possible lymph node involvement will be encountered more frequently. The decision to recommend traditional radical lymphadenectomy may be guided by further limited sampling of lymph nodes. The sentinel lymph node is the first node to receive lymphatic drainage from the primary tumor site and can be considered the first site of micrometastasis along the route of lymphatic drainage. Studies are investigating sentinel lymph node navigation with radiocolloid dye or indocyanine green injected endoscopically,[33,34] or computed tomography lymphography with nanoscale iodized oil emulsion[35] to increase the accuracy of detecting lymph node metastasis.[36] Combined ESD and sentinel node navigation surgery is a feasible, minimally invasive procedure that allows en bloc tumor resection while assessing the pathologic status of the lymph nodes. A case series of combined ESD and sentinel node navigation was conducted in 13 patients with clinical T1 N0 ($\leq$3 cm) EGC.[34] The procedure was converted to gastrectomy in 1 patient after sentinel node navigation surgery. En bloc resection was achieved in all cases, although 2 patients underwent gastrectomy because their lesions had tumor-positive vertical margins.

Endoscopic Full-thickness Resection/Laparoscopic Intragastric Full-thickness Excision

Endoscopic full-thickness resection or laparoscopic intragastric full-thickness excision for EGC has limited indication because of the potential for tumor dissemination into the abdominal space during the procedure. At present, several studies are in various states of publication, and techniques are being developed to accomplish nonexposed endoscopic wall-inversion surgery. This new method may be a viable alternative to surgery in patients who have submucosal tumors with or without ulceration, or mucosal tumors that are technically difficult to resect with ESD.[37–39]

Hybrid Natural Orifice Transluminal Endoscopic Surgery

The rapid evolution of ESD has allowed the procedure to become more widely applied. In addition, new diagnostic and therapeutic techniques have become available. One example is natural orifice transluminal endoscopic surgery (NOTES), in which abdominal operations are performed with an endoscope passed through a natural orifice (eg, mouth, urethra, anus) and then through an internal incision in the stomach, vagina, or colon.[40] This procedure allows the flexible endoscope to reach organs outside the lumen of the bowel. NOTES is minimally invasive compared with open surgery and has fewer risks. EMR or ESD can be combined with laparoscopic or thoracoscopic sentinel node mapping and NOTES to allow endoscopic treatment of gastrointestinal cancers with a risk of lymph node metastasis. Hybrid NOTES for EGC consists of endoscopic full-thickness gastric resection and a laparoscopic lymphadenectomy. A prospective, pilot study of NOTES in 14 patients with EGC has been published by Cho and colleagues[41] in Korea. Hybrid NOTES could be a bridge between endoscopic resection and laparoscopic surgery to avert extensive gastrectomy in patients with EGC.

SUMMARY

ESD improves the quality of life of patients with EGC and dysplasia by preserving gastric function. ESD in the treatment of EGC and dysplasia has become standard treatment in Japan and Korea and is being developed and implemented in many major centers in Asia. With a well-designed prospective study, long-term outcomes of expanded criteria for endoscopic resection of EGC are expected to provide reliable indications for endoscopic treatment. Moreover, ongoing and novel clinical investigations of minimally invasive approaches and close collaboration between Western and Asian countries are expected to establish the best way to treat EGC.

REFERENCES

1. Carter KJ, Schaffer HA, Ritchie WP Jr. Early gastric cancer. Ann Surg 1984; 199(5):604–9.
2. Everett SM, Axon AT. Early gastric cancer in Europe. Gut 1997;41(2):142–50.
3. Takekoshi T, Baba Y, Ota H, et al. Endoscopic resection of early gastric carcinoma: results of a retrospective analysis of 308 cases. Endoscopy 1994;26(4):352–8.
4. Isomoto H, Shikuwa S, Yamaguchi N, et al. Endoscopic submucosal dissection for early gastric cancer: a large-scale feasibility study. Gut 2009;58(3):331–6.
5. Japanese Gastric Cancer Association. Japanese classification of gastric carcinoma - 2nd English edition. Gastric Cancer 1998;1(1):10–24.
6. Yamaguchi N, Isomoto H, Fukuda E, et al. Clinical outcomes of endoscopic submucosal dissection for early gastric cancer by indication criteria. Digestion 2009; 80(3):173–81.
7. Gotoda T, Yanagisawa A, Sasako M, et al. Incidence of lymph node metastasis from early gastric cancer: estimation with a large number of cases at two large centers. Gastric Cancer 2000;3(4):219–25.
8. Kim JJ, Lee JH, Jung HY, et al. EMR for early gastric cancer in Korea: a multi-center retrospective study. Gastrointest Endosc 2007;66(4):693–700.
9. Park YS, Park SW, Kim TI, et al. Endoscopic enucleation of upper-GI submucosal tumors by using an insulated-tip electrosurgical knife. Gastrointest Endosc 2004; 59(3):409–15.
10. Oda I, Saito D, Tada M, et al. A multicenter retrospective study of endoscopic resection for early gastric cancer. Gastric Cancer 2006;9(4):262–70.
11. Oka S, Tanaka S, Kaneko I, et al. Advantage of endoscopic submucosal dissection compared with EMR for early gastric cancer. Gastrointest Endosc 2006;64(6):877–83.
12. Imagawa A, Okada H, Kawahara Y, et al. Endoscopic submucosal dissection for early gastric cancer: results and degrees of technical difficulty as well as success. Endoscopy 2006;38(10):987–90.
13. Chung IK, Lee JH, Lee SH, et al. Therapeutic outcomes in 1000 cases of endoscopic submucosal dissection for early gastric neoplasms: Korean ESD Study Group multicenter study. Gastrointest Endosc 2009;69(69):1228–35.
14. Jung HY. Endoscopic resection for early gastric cancer: current status in Korea. Dig Endosc 2012;24(Suppl 1):159–65.
15. Jang JS, Choi SR, Qureshi W, et al. Long-term outcomes of endoscopic submucosal dissection in gastric neoplastic lesions at a single institution in South Korea. Scand J Gastroenterol 2009;44(11):1315–22.
16. Min BH, Lee JH, Kim JJ, et al. Clinical outcomes of endoscopic submucosal dissection (ESD) for treating early gastric cancer: comparison with endoscopic mucosal resection after circumferential precutting (EMR-P). Dig Liver Dis 2009; 41(3):201–9.
17. Chang CC, Lee IL, Chen PJ, et al. Endoscopic submucosal dissection for gastric epithelial tumors: a multicenter study in Taiwan. J Formos Med Assoc 2009; 108(1):38–44.

18. Lian J, Chen S, Zhang Y, et al. A meta-analysis of endoscopic submucosal dissection and EMR for early gastric cancer. Gastrointest Endosc 2012;76(4): 763–70.

19. Goto O, Fujishiro M, Kodashima S, et al. Outcomes of endoscopic submucosal dissection for early gastric cancer with special reference to validation for curability criteria. Endoscopy 2009;41(2):118–22.

20. Nakamoto S, Sakai Y, Kasanuki J, et al. Indications for the use of endoscopic mucosal resection for early gastric cancer in Japan: a comparative study with endoscopic submucosal dissection. Endoscopy 2009;41(9):746–50.

21. Choi KS, Jung HY, Choi KD, et al. EMR versus gastrectomy for intramucosal gastric cancer: comparison of long-term outcomes. Gastrointest Endosc 2011; 73(5):942–8.

22. Ahn JY, Jung HY, Choi KD, et al. Endoscopic and oncologic outcomes after endoscopic resection for early gastric cancer: 1370 cases of absolute and extended indications. Gastrointest Endosc 2011;74(3):485–93.

23. Nagano H, Ohyama S, Fukunaga T, et al. Indications for gastrectomy after incomplete EMR for early gastric cancer. Gastric Cancer 2005;8(3):149–54.

24. Ryu KW, Choi IJ, Doh YW, et al. Surgical indication for non-curative endoscopic resection in early gastric cancer. Ann Surg Oncol 2007;14(12):3428–34.

25. An JY, Baik YH, Choi MG, et al. Predictive factors for lymph node metastasis in early gastric cancer with submucosal invasion: analysis of a single institutional experience. Ann Surg 2007;246(5):749–53.

26. Lee JH, Kim JH, Kim DH, et al. Is surgical treatment necessary after non-curative endoscopic resection for early gastric cancer? J Gastric Cancer 2010;10(4): 182–7.

27. Abe N, Takeuchi H, Ohki A, et al. Long-term outcomes of combination of endoscopic submucosal dissection and laparoscopic lymph node dissection without gastrectomy for early gastric cancer patients who have a potential risk of lymph node metastasis. Gastrointest Endosc 2011;74(4):792–7.

28. Kamada K, Tomatsuri N, Yoshida N. Endoscopic submucosal dissection for undifferentiated early gastric cancer as the expanded indication lesion. Digestion 2012;85(2):111–5.

29. Kunisaki C, Takahashi M, Nagahori Y, et al. Risk factors for lymph node metastasis in histologically poorly differentiated type early gastric cancer. Endoscopy 2009;41(6):498–503.

30. Park YD, Chung YJ, Chung HY, et al. Factors related to lymph node metastasis and the feasibility of endoscopic mucosal resection for treating poorly differentiated adenocarcinoma of the stomach. Endoscopy 2008;40(1):7–10.

31. Park JM, Kim SW, Nam KW, et al. Is it reasonable to treat early gastric cancer with signet ring cell histology by endoscopic resection? Analysis of factors related to lymph-node metastasis. Eur J Gastroenterol Hepatol 2009;21(10):1132–5.

32. Goh PG, Jeong HY, Kim MJ, et al. Clinical outcomes of endoscopic submucosal dissection for undifferentiated or submucosal invasive early gastric cancer. Clin Endosc 2011;44(2):116–22.

33. Kelder W, Nimura H, Takahashi N, et al. Sentinel node mapping with indocyanine green (ICG) and infrared ray detection in early gastric cancer: an accurate method that enables a limited lymphadenectomy. Eur J Surg Oncol 2010;36(6): 552–8.

34. Bok GH, Kim YJ, Jin SY, et al. Endoscopic submucosal dissection with sentinel node navigation surgery for early gastric cancer. Endoscopy 2012;44(10): 953–6.

35. Lim JS, Choi J, Song J, et al. Nanoscale iodized oil emulsion: a useful tracer for pretreatment sentinel node detection using CT lymphography in a normal canine gastric model. Surg Endosc 2012;26(8):2267–74.

36. Takeuchi H, Kitagawa Y. New sentinel node mapping technologies for early gastric cancer. Ann Surg Oncol 2013;20(2):522–32.

37. Goto O, Mitsui T, Fujishiro M, et al. New method of endoscopic full-thickness resection: a pilot study of non-exposed endoscopic wall-inversion surgery in an ex vivo porcine model. Gastric Cancer 2011;14(2):183–7.

38. Hoya Y, Yamashita M, Sasaki T, et al. Laparoscopic intragastric full-thickness excision (LIFE) of early gastric cancer under flexible endoscopic control–introduction of new technique using animal. Surg Laparosc Endosc Percutan Tech 2007;17(2):111–5.

39. Inoue H, Ikeda H, Hosoya T, et al. Endoscopic mucosal resection, endoscopic submucosal dissection, and beyond: full-layer resection for gastric cancer with nonexposure technique (CLEAN-NET). Surg Oncol Clin N Am 2012;21(1):129–40.

40. Chun HJ, Keum B, Park S. The current status of natural orifice transluminal endoscopic surgery (NOTES). Korean J Gastrointest Endosc 2009;38(3):121–7 [in Korean].

41. Cho WY, Kim YJ, Cho JY, et al. Hybrid natural orifice transluminal endoscopic surgery: endoscopic full-thickness resection of early gastric cancer and laparoscopic regional lymph node dissection–14 human cases. Endoscopy 2011; 43(2):134–9.

ESD Around the World: Europe

Horst Neuhaus, MD

KEYWORDS

- Endoscopic submucosal dissection • Endoscopic mucosal resection
- Early gastric carcinoma • Early esophageal carcinoma • Early colorectal neoplasia

KEY POINTS

- Clinical experience and level of evidence of endoscopic submucosal dissection (ESD) are still limited in Europe.
- Excellent data from Asia cannot be reproduced; promising data were reported from centers with a higher case volume.
- Poor results of ESD have to be considered at the beginning of the learning curve.
- ESD is clearly indicated in selected patients with early gastric cancer and early esophageal squamous carcinoma.
- There seems to be no advantage of ESD over endoscopic mucosal resection in terms of clinical outcome in cases with early Barrett neoplasia and early colorectal neoplasia; potential niche indications need further evaluation.
- Structured training programs and enrollment of patients in well-designed trials are strongly needed.

INTRODUCTION

Endoscopic resection of early gastrointestinal neoplasia offers advantages over surgery with respect to organ preservation, safety, and cost-effectiveness. However, the local approach requires that the risk of lymph node metastasis is very low and recurrence of neoplasia is rare or endoscopically manageable.

Grading of neoplasia and the depth of vertical invasion are the most important predictive parameters for lymph node metastasis, with variations with regard to the site in the gastrointestinal tract.[1–3] Even advanced endoscopic imaging frequently does not allow accurate preoperative determination of the vertical invasion of early neoplastic lesions. Detailed analysis and classification of the mucosal structure and the microvascular architecture has proved to be accurate according to Japanese studies, but it remains unclear whether these results can be reproduced in Europe because of the limited experience in interpretation of detailed findings and infrequent use of

Disclosure: Technical support came from ERBE Elektromedizin GmbH, Tübingen, for the evaluation of WESD.

Department of Internal Medicine, Evangelisches Krankenhaus Düsseldorf, Teaching Hospital of the University of Düsseldorf, Kirchfeldstrasse 40, Düsseldorf 40217, Germany
E-mail address: horst.neuhaus@evk-duesseldorf.de

Gastrointest Endoscopy Clin N Am 24 (2014) 295–311
http://dx.doi.org/10.1016/j.giec.2013.11.002
1052-5157/14/$ – see front matter © 2014 Elsevier Inc. All rights reserved.

magnifying endoscopy.[4,5] Endoscopic ultrasonography (EUS) seems to be valuable for identifying early gastric cancers that meet the expanded-indication criteria for endoscopic submucosal dissection (ESD) in Japan.[6] On the other hand, a retrospective cohort study from Amsterdam in the Netherlands indicated that EUS has no clinical impact on the workup of early esophageal neoplasia.[7]

In Europe, it is therefore widely accepted that endoscopic resection is an appropriate diagnostic approach to obtain specimens for accurate histopathologic evaluation, which may change grading and local staging of early neoplasia determined by prior biopsies and imaging. It allows the identification of more advanced tumor stages in patients for whom surgery is required because the risks of incomplete resection or lymph node metastasis outweigh the disadvantages of a major operation. The aim is, however, to achieve curative resection, preferably in an en bloc fashion, to confirm vertical and horizontal tumor-free margins (R0 resection) by histology. Piecemeal resection usually allows determination of the vertical invasion, thus allowing patients with an increased risk of lymph node metastasis to be identified. However, horizontal tumor-free margins cannot be evaluated by examination of several specimens (R1 resection horizontal margins). Even in cases of endoscopically complete resection, the risk of residual neoplasia and local recurrence remains indeterminate in these cases. Therefore, piecemeal resection requires close follow-up examinations, for example, every 3 months within the first year. Residual tumors after piecemeal resection are usually small and can be easily removed. In contrast to the problem of residual neoplasia, true recurrences after complete remission are probably rare and have to be differentiated from metachronous lesions.

Conventional resection is performed as endoscopic mucosal resection (EMR) by snare wiring, which usually does not allow resection of mucosal neoplastic lesions larger than 1 to 2 cm in diameter in a single piece. En bloc resection can even fail in cases of smaller lesions depending on their location and shape. Therefore, extension of EMR frequently has to be performed in a piecemeal fashion. In contrast to EMR, the technique of ESD allows resection of even large lesions in a single piece. In Japan and other Asian countries, ESD has become the treatment of choice for early gastric cancer and is increasingly also used for early esophageal and colorectal neoplasia. Two recent meta-analyses demonstrated significantly higher rates of en bloc resection and curative resection for ESD in comparison with EMR.[8,9] On the other hand, ESD was more time-consuming and had higher rates of complications, mainly related to perforation and bleeding. All of the included controlled studies were performed in Asia except a single small trial from Italy.[10] The quality of many of these trials is limited in terms of design and lack of intention-to-treat analyses, and the duration of follow-up was even not recorded in some of the series. Therefore, the level of evidence of the clinical value of ESD is still limited and mainly based on data from Japan, which may not be directly applicable to Europe, in particular with respect to oncologic and procedural parameters. Outcome of ESD may be less favorable because of the limited Western expertise in this challenging and potentially hazardous technique. The potential advantages have to be carefully balanced against the pros and cons of well-established EMR techniques and surgery in more advanced stages. In this context, the current role of ESD in Europe must be differentiated with respect to the biology and site of early neoplasia in the gastrointestinal tract.

DEFINITION OF OUTCOME PARAMETERS OF ENDOSCOPIC RESECTION

The comparison between a large number of published trials on EMR and ESD remains difficult because of different criteria for selection of patients and definition of outcome parameters. Common terms are shown in **Box 1**. Some such terms seem to be used differently in Eastern and Western publications. "Curative resection" is rarely reported in European trials, but the definition even varies in Japanese reports. It usually includes histologically complete resection of any kind of neoplasia. However, this term was restricted to cancer in a large study of ESD of colorectal neoplasia, which means that the resection could have been "curative" despite remnants of adenoma.[11] On the other hand, the terms "complete remission" or "complete local remission" have been defined in Europe, in particular for EMR of early Barrett neoplasia, but are uncommon in Japan.

Studies on endoscopic resection also vary in definition and registration of complications. In contrast to publications on surgical procedures, the 30-day morbidity and mortality rates are rarely reported. Reports on further follow-up rarely differentiate between residual, recurrent, and metachronous neoplasia. A residual neoplasia can be explained by incomplete resection, whereas recurrences may be less frequent than reported and may have an oncologic background similar to that of metachronous lesions.

There are also well-known regional differences between histopathologic diagnoses of some gastrointestinal neoplasms, mainly depending on cytologic criteria combined with atypical architecture in the East, in contrast to architectural and anatomic criteria in the West. As an example, the Japanese definition of "intramucosal cancer" in the colorectum corresponds to "high-grade dysplasia," which is the term mainly used in the United States, and "high-grade intraepithelial neoplasia" in reports from Europe. The European terminology corresponds to the classification of the World Health Organization (WHO).[12] In contrast to those of the upper gastrointestinal tract, these lesions have no risk of lymph node metastasis.

ESD OF EARLY GASTRIC NEOPLASIA

Early gastric neoplasia includes adenoma and cancer limited to the mucosa or submucosa, irrespective of the presence of lymph node metastasis. Endoscopic treatment should be restricted to patients with no risk of lymph node metastasis. Its prediction

---

Box 1
Outcome parameters for endoscopic resection of early gastrointestinal neoplasia

En bloc resection

  Resection in a single piece without fragmentation (endoscopic assessment)

R0 resection

  Lateral and vertical margins free of neoplasia (histologic assessment)

Curative resection

  R0 resection and

    No lymphatic or venous infiltration

    No undifferentiated areas

Complete local remission

  R0 + 1 negative follow-up endoscopy

  R0 vertical/R1 horizontal + at least 1 negative follow-up endoscopy

requires a detailed histopathologic analysis of the specimen, which can only be provided after en bloc resection. Piecemeal resection may miss small areas with deeper invasion or invasion of lymphatic vessels. Indications restricted to the standard criteria according the Japanese Gastric Cancer Association (JGCA) have been also accepted for a curative approach in many European countries, and are part of the German Guidelines on the management of gastric cancer.[2,13–15] By contrast, the expanded criteria of the JGCA are so far not considered as appropriate indications for endoscopic resection.[15] ESD can be considered if patients have an increased risk for surgery or are enrolled in appropriate clinical trials. The decision making should be discussed in tumor boards.

There are several reasons for the limitation of indications in Europe. The current definition of the expanded criteria is mainly based on the histopathologic analysis of the rate of lymph node metastases in gastrectomy specimens of patients with different stages of early gastric cancer in Japan.[2] It remains undetermined as to whether these results can be applied to Western countries, owing to the lack of appropriate trials. A single study from Germany indicated that endoscopic resection of gastric carcinoma with deep infiltration of the mucosa (m3) or superficial invasion of the submucosa (sm1) is associated with a risk of lymph node metastases of 13% and 21%, respectively.[16] However, most of these cases were undifferentiated cancers, which do not meet the extended criteria. Several Japanese studies showed that en bloc resection rates were significantly higher in the guideline group than in the expanded group, but overall survival was statistically not different.[13,17–19] These results have to be confirmed in Europe, but this remains difficult because of the limited number of detected cases with early gastric neoplasia.

The number of European prospective case series or feasibility trials on gastric ESD is limited (**Table 1**). Only a few studies have included more than a single center. The author's group participated in the first European clinical trial on ESD, which included esophageal, gastric, and duodenal mucosal neoplasia and submucosal tumors in a total of 37 patients from 2 centers.[20] En bloc resection was achieved in only 54% of mucosal lesions and 50% of submucosal tumors, with a total R0 resection rate of 37%. No severe complications that necessitated surgery or caused major morbidity occurred.

The author's group subsequently evaluated a multibending double-channel endoscope (R-scope) in anesthetized pigs. After promising results, 10 patients with early gastric carcinoma were included in a clinical feasibility trial involving 6 European centers.[21] En bloc resection was achieved in 6 cases. Complications were registered in half of the patients, and surgery became necessary in 2 cases because of early and delayed perforation. The use of this complex endoscope was difficult, and it seemed not to be superior to standard instruments in combination with accessories used in Japanese series.

Furthers trials were designed as prospective case reports from single centers with limited numbers of operating endoscopists (see **Table 1**). In a Portuguese study, ESD performed by a single endoscopist with an insulated-tip knife achieved a 79% en bloc resection rate in 19 patients with early gastric neoplasia.[22] The higher R0 resection rate of 89% is due to the surprising result that histopathology confirmed in 4 cases that "both lateral and vertical margins were free of lesions (R0)" despite piecemeal resection. No perforations and one major bleed were registered. Only one case of recurrence was observed within a median follow-up period of 10 months. An Italian single-center study reported on ESD with an insulated-tip knife in 12 patients with early gastric cancer.[10] Curative resection was achieved in 92% of these cases, with complications in 16%, and no recurrence during a mean follow-up of 31 months.

Table 1
European case series and feasibility trials on ESD

Authors,[Ref.] Year	No. of Centers	ESD Site/Patients (n)				Resection Success (%)		Mean Procedure Time (min)	Complication Rate (%)	Recurrence Rate (%)	Mean Follow-Up (mo)
		E	S	D	CR	En Bloc	R0				
Rösch et al,[20] 2004	2	12	24	1	—	53	37	—	17	—	—
Neuhaus et al,[21] 2009	6	—	10	—	—	60	50	87	50	—	—
Dinis-Ribeiro et al,[22] 2009	1	—	19	—	—	79	89	90	5	5	10
Catalano et al,[10] 2009	1	—	12	—	—	92	92	111	16	0	31
Coda et al,[23] 2010	1	3	7	1	14	84	100	120	32	8	18
Probst et al,[25] 2009	1	—	91	—	—	87	74	157	9	6	27
Schumacher et al,[26] 2012	1	—	29	—	—	90	64	74	14	10	22
Farhat et al,[31] 2011	16	27	75	1	72	77	73	105	29	—	—
Repici et al,[38] 2010	1	20	—	—	—	100	90	89	15	0	18
Neuhaus et al,[44] 2012	1	30	—	—	—	90	39	75	7	96	17
Probst et al,[49] 2012	1	—	—	—	82	82	70	176	9	9	24
Repici et al,[50] 2013	1	—	—	—	40	90	80	86	8	3	12

Abbreviations: CR, colorectum; D, duodenum; E, esophagus; S, stomach.

One patient had to undergo surgery for management of gastric perforation. Another Italian feasibility trial reported on excellent results of ESD in various sites of the gastrointestinal tract including 7 gastric lesions.[23] In Germany, a tertiary referral center performed ESD with various types of knives in 71 patients with mucosal or submucosal lesions located in various sites of the gastrointestinal tract, including 51 early gastric neoplasias.[24] En bloc resection rates and R0 resection rates were 77.1% and 65.7%, respectively, in the first half of the study, and increased to 86.1% and 72.2%, respectively, in the second half. No recurrence was observed after R0 en bloc resection. Two of 4 perforations required surgical treatment at the beginning of the learning curve. The same group recently reported on the largest European single-center trial on ESD of early gastric neoplasia (see **Table 1**).[25] Over a period of 7 years, 91 patients underwent ESD by 2 endoscopists, and achieved an en bloc resection rate of 74%. According to the study period and the inclusion criteria, 51 of these patients had been obviously already included in the previous trial of the same group on collected data on ESD.[24] Only 17% of the 66 cases with early gastric carcinoma met the standard guideline criteria, which indicates that even in specialized centers most patients have more advanced tumor stages and have to be enrolled in trials according to German guidelines. The R0 resection rates for adenomas, guideline criteria, and expanded criteria of early gastric cancers were 79%, 69%, and 90%, respectively. No perforation occurred during any of the procedures. The overall complication rate was 9.4%, and there was no mortality. All complications were endoscopically managed. The success rates improved over the study period, but the mean procedural time of approximately 2.5 hours remained unchanged with consideration of inclusion of an increasing number of larger lesions. The recurrence rate of early gastric carcinoma was 5.6% over a mean follow-up period of 27 months.

The author's group recently reported on the first clinical trial of water-jet–assisted ESD (WESD) technology in patients with early gastric neoplasia.[26] This system allows pressure-controlled injection of fluids through the tip of the recently developed Hybrid-Knife (ERBE Elektromedizin GmbH, Tübingen, Germany). Submucosal injection, circumferential cutting and dissection of lesions, and coagulation of bleeding sources can be performed with the same device without the need to change the instrument. These options should accelerate the procedure, and may increase its safety and efficacy (**Fig. 1**). Experimental trials in both ex vivo and in vivo pig models showed that the gastrointestinal mucosa of different sites can be effectively and safely lifted by placement of the HybridKnife on the wall and needleless injection of saline solution with pressures between 30 and 70 bar.[27–29] The prospective clinical study included 29 patients with early gastric neoplasia in whom this new ESD technology achieved en bloc resection in 90% of the cases, with a median time of 74 minutes. Intraprocedural bleedings and small perforations in 11 and 3 cases, respectively, were able to be managed conservatively. The 30-day morbidity rate was 13.8%, because of postoperative pain in 3 cases and delayed bleeding in 1 case. There was no need for surgery for management of complications. A 93-year-old patient died the night after WESD without evidence of a procedure-related complication. Histopathology demonstrated an R0 resection rate of 64%. With a single exception, all resections achieved vertical neoplasia-free tumor margins. Three recurrences were registered within a median follow-up period of 22 months. One of these was endoscopically resected; 2 patients underwent surgery.

Together with a large referral center in Shanghai, the author's group recently performed the first randomized controlled trial in 109 patients with early gastric neoplasia for comparison of WESD with conventional ESD.[30] There were no significant differences with regard to resection rates or complications, but WESD was significantly

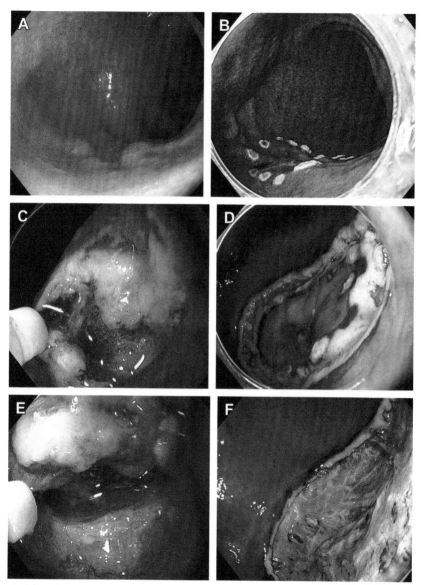

Fig. 1. (*A*) Early gastric cancer (types 0–IIa and IIc) at the greater curvature. (*B*) Narrow-band imaging shows coagulation markers placed at the periphery of the tumor with a safety margin of 5 mm. (*C*) Circumferential incision alongside the periphery of the markers by use of a water-jet–assisted HybridKnife, allowing alternating submucosal infiltration of saline solution mixed with indicarmine and cutting without changing the device. (*D*) Complete circumferential incision of the lesion. (*E*) Dissection of deeper layers of the submucosa, which can be easily identified according to the bluish color and appropriate distance to the muscle layer at 6 o'clock and the lesion at 12 o'clock. (*F*) Area after en bloc resection. (*G*) Resected specimen appropriate for a detailed histopathologic evaluation.

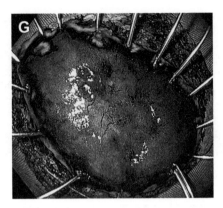

Fig. 1. (*continued*)

faster than conventional ESD and required fewer changes of accessories. Details of this study have not yet been published.

A multi-institutional report collected case series on ESD in various sites of the gastrointestinal tract from 16 centers in France (see **Table 1**).[31] Most of the 188 included patients had neoplastic lesions in the stomach (n = 75) and colorectum (n = 85). Gastric ESD achieved en bloc and R0 resection rates of 85.3% and 84.0%, respectively. Perforation occurred in 34 of all 188 patients (18.1%), and required surgical treatment in 17.6% of these cases. All of the 21 clinically significant bleedings were able to be managed endoscopically or required only observation. There was no significant difference in complication rates between the first and second halves of the study in the 3 centers that enrolled more than 30 cases. Follow-up data on residual or recurrent neoplasia were not reported.

A survey among European endoscopists who published in highly demanding medical journals clearly indicates that gastric ESD is still not a common practice.[32] Only 20 centers provided data on gastric ESD, mainly performed by a single endoscopist. Each one treated a mean number of only 4 cases during the last year of the survey, with a total number of 510 ESD cases. Histologically confirmed en bloc resection of early gastric neoplasia was achieved in 78% of all cases with an R0 resection rate of 77%. The rate of major complications was 13%. The investigators concluded that European gastroenterologists are still beginners in performing ESD, but that they achieve a high rate of efficacy. The procedure-related morbidity appears to be higher than in most Japanese series, but the investigators assume that proper training could probably reduce it. It is not known whether these data are still representative for European endoscopists.

ESD OF EARLY ESOPHAGEAL NEOPLASIA

ESD has been increasingly accepted for the treatment of early squamous cell carcinoma of the esophagus in Asian countries. Histopathologic evaluation of surgically resected specimens indicates that the risk of lymph node metastases is extremely low if the cancer is limited to the superficial and mid layer of the mucosa (m1 and m2).[1,33] Several Japanese trials have demonstrated that ESD achieves complete resection of these highly selected cases, which is required for a detailed histopathology of the specimen and avoidance of local tumor recurrence.[34–36] In Europe, squamous cell carcinoma is rarely detected in these early stages, probably because of a lack of screening gastroscopy and limited experience in endoscopic evaluation of the related minimal mucosal changes. In addition, the esophagus is one of the most difficult sites for ESD, which should be limited to endoscopists with appropriate experience in gastric and/or rectal ESD (**Fig. 2**).[37] These reasons may explain why only a single prospective case series on ESD of early esophageal squamous cell carcinoma was reported (see **Table 1**).[38] The procedure was performed in 20 patients who were included over a study period of 3 years. En bloc resection was achieved in all cases, with a mean time of 1.5 hours. None of the 18 patients with R0 resection had residual or recurrent cancer during a mean follow-up of 18 months. ESD caused one symptomatic esophageal stricture. No other clinically relevant complications were observed.

In Europe, Barrett adenocarcinoma is by far the most frequent type of esophageal cancer detected at an early stage. EMR has been widely accepted for local treatment of high-grade intraepithelial neoplasia (HGIN) and mucosal adenocarcinoma. This approach has been extensively studied in several European centers.[39,40] Focal EMR achieves complete local remission of neoplasia in 97% to 99% of cases, and severe complications rarely occur. The frequent problem of recurrent or metachronous neoplastic lesions seems to be avoidable by the safe and effective combination of EMR with radiofrequency ablation (RFA), according to recent and ongoing trials.[41] In view of these excellent results, it will be difficult to show advantages of ESD over EMR, particularly as ESD is such a time-consuming, technically demanding, and potentially hazardous technique.

Widespread ESD seems to allow complete eradication of neoplastic and nonneoplastic Barrett epithelium with the objectives of achieving R0 resection and minimizing the risk of recurrence.[42] However, this approach frequently causes severe esophageal stricture to an extent comparable with stepwise radical EMR, which is inferior to a combination of EMR with RFA regarding this type of complication.[43] The author's group[44] performed the first prospective clinical trial on ESD in 30 patients with early Barrett neoplasia. The primary objective of the study was to achieve en bloc resection of mucosal neoplasia (see **Table 1**). En bloc resection, and even more so, R0 resection, can rarely be obtained by EMR, but may allow a more precise histopathologic evaluation and promise a decreased risk of residual neoplasia. WESD achieved complete resection and en bloc resection in 96.7% and 90%, respectively. No complications were observed except for 2 minor bleedings. R0 resection could be confirmed in only 10 of the 26 patients (38.5%) with HGIN or adenocarcinoma. This disappointing result seems to be related mainly to inappropriate delineation and preoperative marking of the lateral tumor margins, which can be difficult especially in the flat lesions of Barrett esophagus. The rate of complete remission of neoplasia was 96.6% with a mean follow-up of 17 months. Additional RFA was performed in 10 patients to eradicate residual nonneoplastic Barrett epithelium. This promising outcome was achieved by a single session of WESD, and has to be balanced against comparable results after piecemeal EMR, which sometimes has to be repeated. The author recently discussed the potential role of ESD in early Barrett neoplasia in detail, and initiated a prospective randomized controlled trial to compare ESD with EMR in this setting.[44]

ESD OF EARLY COLORECTAL NEOPLASIA

Numerous Western studies have demonstrated that EMR is effective and safe for curative treatment of large sessile or flat colorectal adenomas or lateral spreading tumors (LSTs).[45–47] EMR frequently has to be performed in a piecemeal fashion, but histology usually allows the identification of cases with adenocarcinoma and those patients who have to undergo surgery because of submucosal infiltration. Predictive

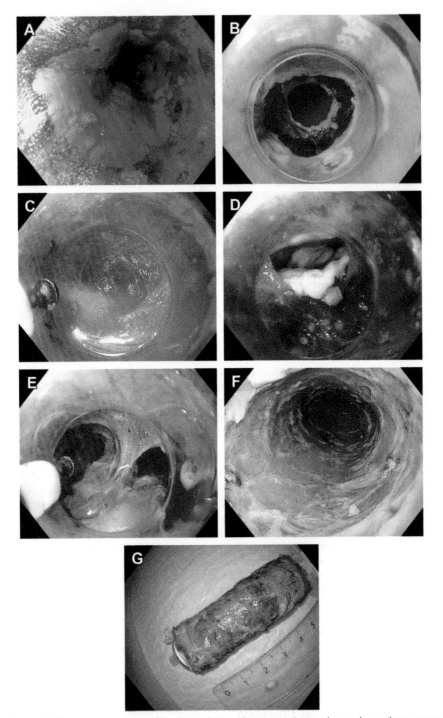

Fig. 2. (*A*) Chomoendoscopy with iodine solution demonstrating early esophageal squamous cell carcinoma (type 0–IIb) with circumferential extension over a distance of 7 cm. (*B*) Circumferential incision of the mucosa below the markers of the distal tumor margin. (*C*) Tunneling of the submucosa between the mucosa at 12 o'clock and the circular muscle layer at 6 o'clock from the proximal to the distal tumor margins. (*D*) The first tunnel approaches the distal mucosal incision. (*E*) Dissection of the tissue between the first and second submucosal tunnel located at the contralateral site. (*F*) Resection area after en bloc endoscopic submucosal dissection (ESD) over a longitudinal distance of 9 cm. (*G*) Tubular specimen stretched on a syringe.

factors of submucosal cancers that should be considered before EMR are nongranular LSTs, lesions classified as Paris type 0-IIc or 0-IIa and IIc, and/or those with Pit Pattern type V.[46] Risk factors for failure of a complete removal of lesions in a single session are the nonlifting sign, involvement of the ileocecal valve, previous attempts of removal, and/or a difficult position.[48] The risk of perforation is very low, and intraprocedural or delayed bleedings can be endoscopically managed or stop spontaneously. The main disadvantage of piecemeal EMR is related to the high rate (20%–30%) of residual or recurrent adenoma. However, short-term follow-up colonoscopies allow detection and definitive resection or ablation of these lesions in most cases.[46] Predictive parameters for residual neoplasia after EMR are piecemeal resection, histologically incomplete resection, and components of high-grade dysplasia.[45,48]

In Japan, ESD has been increasingly accepted for endoscopic treatment of selected patients with early colorectal neoplasia. The selection criteria consider parameters predictive of an increased risk of submucosal cancer and failures of EMR. The aim is en bloc resection to allow a detailed histopathologic evaluation and to minimize the rate of residual neoplasia. A recent Japanese multicenter trial on ESD of colorectal neoplasia was performed in 1111 patients who met at least 1 of the following inclusion criteria: nongranular type LST larger than 20 mm or granular type LST larger than 30 mm in diameter, large villous tumors, as well as intramucosal lesions, recurrent lesions, and residual mucosal lesions that showed a nonlifting sign.[11] The high en bloc resection rate of 88% in this trial has to be outweighed against the technical difficulties and long duration of the procedure (average of 116 minutes) and a perforation rate of 5%. In comparison with piecemeal EMR, patients with lesions limited to the mucosa probably do not benefit from a more detailed histology provided by en bloc resection, because there is no risk of lymph node metastasis even in those with high-grade intraepithelial neoplasia or "mucosal cancer." Deeper invasion into the submucosa can also be diagnosed by piecemeal resection. From an oncologic perspective, a clinically relevant advantage of ESD seems to be limited to patients with submucosal invasion of differentiated cancer of less than 1 mm.[3] R0 resection is required to consider endoscopic resection as a curative treatment. However, only 10% of the patients in the Japanese trial met these criteria. In contrast to this limited impact on clinical outcome, a major advantage of ESD of colorectal lesions is a low recurrence rate of approximately 2%, which is substantially lower than that of EMR. This low rate may allow extension between follow-up intervals and the avoidance of reintervention for removal of residual neoplasia.

According to the aforementioned French multi-institutional report on collected case series of ESD, the colorectum seems to be the most frequently approached site.[31] With regard to the less obvious oncologic advantages over EMR compared with gastric neoplasia, the main reasons for the relatively frequent use, in particular of rectal ESD, is probably due to the technically easy approach and management of potential complications. Despite the lower threshold to perform colorectal ESD and the high volume of cases in Europe, so far only 2 prospective single-center cases have been published (see **Table 1**).[49,50] A large German referral center included 82 patients with large sessile lesions in the rectum (87%) and sigmoid (13%) (see **Table 1**).[49] Similarly to its recent report on gastric ESD, some of these patients had been obviously already included in a previous trial on ESD in different sites of the gastrointestinal tract, with an overlap of more than half of the study period.[24] The inclusion criteria were adjusted to Japanese recommendations. The rates for successful ESD, en bloc, and R0 resection were 92.7%, 81.6%, and 69.7%, respectively. The R0 resection rates significantly increased and the procedural duration decreased with experience during the study period. Resection was incomplete in 13 of 14 resected cancers, so that additional surgery was recommended. Therefore, this trial showed no benefit of ESD in patients with early carcinoma in terms of clinical outcome. Perforation and bleeding were registered in 1.3% and 7.9% of the patients. None of these complications required surgical intervention. During a median period of 23.6 months, follow-up endoscopies revealed residual neoplasia in 6 of 65 patients. The risk was significantly higher after piecemeal resection compared with en bloc resection (41.7% vs 0%). The high rate of residual neoplasia after failure of en bloc resection may indicate that there is no advantage of ESD over EMR if resection in a single piece cannot be achieved. An Italian pilot study enrolled 40 patients with LSTs larger than 3 cm in diameter for WESD.[50] En bloc resection succeeded in 90% of the cases, and failures successfully underwent piecemeal resection. The R0 resection rate was 80%. Histopathology of the resected specimen showed cancer with submucosal invasion in 2 cases. R0 resection had failed in both of these, and surgery was required. Perforation in 1 case and delayed bleeding in 2 cases was able to be managed endoscopically. Only one patient, in whom R0 resection had not been achieved, had residual neoplasia at follow-up endoscopies.

TRAINING FOR ESD IN EUROPE

A panel of experts recently reported consensus statements on ESD in Europe.[37] ESD should meet quality standards, should be performed following national or European Society of Gastrointestinal Endoscopy guidelines or under approval of the Institutional Review Board (IRB), and all cases should be prospectively registered. The panel recommends structured training courses followed by a stepwise clinical approach, starting with ESD in the rectum, then in the distal stomach, colon, proximal stomach, and finally the esophagus. Beginners of ESD probably benefit from training courses including simulators and ex vivo models.[51] Trainees can learn important technical details of the procedure, but there are limitations, in particular with respect to management of complications (eg, intraprocedural bleeding). Therefore, this initial training should be followed by in vivo courses (eg, on anesthetized pigs, which are offered in several European institutions).[52] This kind of training allows determination of various quality parameters (eg, success, procedural duration, and occurrence and management of complications).

After achievement of the appropriate skills ESD can be considered in well-selected patients, but should be performed under supervision of an expert. In contrast to Japan, not the stomach but the rectum is suggested as the initial target organ for clinical training. The main reason is obviously that the case volume of early rectal neoplasia is much higher than that of gastric neoplasia in Western countries. It remains undetermined as to whether this approach is justified, because most rectal lesions are benign LSTs that can be safely and easily removed by the well-established piecemeal EMR. The esophagus could be another organ for appropriate training of ESD in Western countries, in view of the high volume of patients with early Barrett neoplasia. However, ESD is substantially more difficult in the esophagus than in the stomach, because of the challenging anatomy and frequently associated fibrosis and scar formation caused by inflammation in patients with gastroesophageal reflux disease.

SUMMARY

Meta-analyses of controlled trials indicate that ESD is superior to well-established EMR techniques with respect to en bloc resection and curative resection of selected cases of early gastrointestinal neoplasia. However, all but one of these analyzed trials were performed in Asian countries, mainly in patients with early gastric carcinoma, and the quality of most of them is limited. It is questionable whether the results can be applied to Europe with regard to oncologic parameters and results of ESD predominantly performed by endoscopists with limited experience with this difficult and potentially hazardous procedure. According to the few European case series and feasibility trials on ESD, excellent results from Japan cannot be reproduced with regard to success and complication rates as well as procedural duration. Promising data were reported from centers with a higher case volume, in particular for ESD of early gastric cancer. Inappropriate results and unacceptably high complication rates have to be considered when ESD is infrequently performed by endoscopists with limited expertise.

There are no European data on long-term outcomes after ESD and its cost-effectiveness, which will be affected by an average procedural duration of 1.5 to 2 hours and the high costs of the various accessories required. Despite these limitations, ESD should be considered as the method of choice for endoscopic resection in selected patients with early gastric cancer and esophageal squamous cell carcinoma. From an oncologic perspective, it is mandatory in these cases to achieve R0 resection for a complete histopathologic evaluation to minimize the risk of lymph node metastasis. By contrast, there is no proof that ESD is superior to EMR in patients with early Barrett neoplasia. There may be a niche indication in cases with suspicion of submucosal tumor invasion to allow a complete histopathologic evaluation of an en bloc

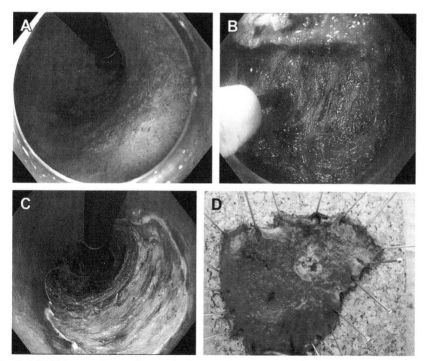

Fig. 3. (A) Widespread sporadic rectal adenoma in a patient with ulcerative colitis; nonlifting after submucosal injection, owing to intensive fibrosis, preventing EMR techniques. (B) Careful dissection of the submucosa and the fibrotic tissue after instillation of saline solution using high pressure of the water-jet–assisted ESD technique. (C) Area after en bloc resection. (D) Resected specimen stretched on cork; histopathology showed adenoma with areas of high-grade intraepithelial neoplasia.

resected specimen. ESD of colorectal lesions seems to be attractive in Europe because of the high case volume and easy access, in particular to rectal early neoplasia. However, the suggested oncologic advantage over EMR has not been shown in the few published reports. Nearly all patients with early colorectal carcinoma had to undergo surgery after ESD because of incomplete resection or histopathologic parameters. In this context, it has to be considered that mucosal cancers in Japan are classified as HGIN according to WHO criteria; they are not associated with any risk of lymph node metastasis, so that easy and fast piecemeal EMR techniques are appropriate according to well-designed prospective trials. The argument of a lower recurrence rate after ESD has to be balanced against the long duration and the risk of this procedure, and the well demonstrated, easy endoscopic management of residual neoplasia. A niche indication for colorectal ESD is lesions that are difficult to remove by EMR (eg, nongranular type LST and recurrent neoplasia with scars after previous resection, or colorectal lesions in inflammatory bowel disease) (**Fig. 3**). The dilemma for Western endoscopists is that these cases with the optimal indication are the most difficult to treat. On the other hand, it is questionable from an ethical point of view to perform ESD just for training reasons on lesions that can be well managed by EMR.

There is no doubt that because of its potential advantages the spectrum of indications for ESD could be expanded in Europe, provided that the technique will be simplified and safer. This goal may be achievable by technical improvements and structured training. In view of these open questions and ethical issues, it is doubtful that ESD can be appropriately evaluated by surveys or registries in Europe. The aim should be to demonstrate that results from Japan can be reproduced in countries with a different group of patients and limited endoscopic skill in ESD. To overcome this problem, centers with a high case volume of early gastrointestinal neoplasia should cooperate and initiate prospective, preferably controlled trials on ESD under IRB approval.

REFERENCES

1. Bollschweiler E, Baldus SE, Schröder W, et al. High rate of lymph node metastasis in submucosal esophageal squamous cell carcinomas and adenocarcinomas. Endoscopy 2006;38:149–56.
2. Gotoda T, Yanagisawa A, Sasako M, et al. Incidence of lymph-node metastasis from early gastric cancer: estimation with a large number of cases at two large centers. Gastric Cancer 2000;3:219–25.
3. Kitajima K, Fujimori T, Fujii S, et al. Correlations between lymph node metastasis and depth of submucosal invasion in submucosal invasive colorectal carcinoma: a Japanese collaborative study. J Gastroenterol 2004;39:534–43.
4. Kobayashi Y, Kudo SE, Miyachi H, et al. Clinical usefulness of pit patterns for detecting colonic lesions requiring surgical treatment. Int J Colorectal Dis 2011;26:1531–40.
5. Kaga M, Inoue H, Kudo SE, et al. Microvascular architecture of early esophageal neoplasia. Oncol Rep 2011;26:1063–7.
6. Okada K, Fujisaki J, Kasuga A, et al. Endoscopic ultrasonography is valuable for identifying early gastric cancers meeting expanded-indication criteria for endoscopic submucosal dissection. Surg Endosc 2011;25:841–8.
7. Pouw RE, Heldoorn N, Herrero LA, et al. Do we still need EUS in the workup of patients with early esophageal neoplasia? A retrospective analysis of 131 cases. Gastrointest Endosc 2011;73:662–8.

8. Cao Y, Liao C, Tan A, et al. Meta-analysis of endoscopic submucosal dissection versus endoscopic mucosal resection for tumors of the gastrointestinal tract. Endoscopy 2009;4:751–7.
9. Lian J, Chen S, Zhang Y, et al. A meta-analysis of endoscopic submucosal dissection and EMR for early gastric cancer. Gastrointest Endosc 2012;76:763–70.
10. Catalano F, Trecca A, Rodella L, et al. The modern treatment of early gastric cancer: our experience in an Italian cohort. Surg Endosc 2009;23:1581–6.
11. Saito Y, Uraoka T, Yamaguchi Y, et al. A prospective, multicenter study of 1111 colorectal endoscopic submucosal dissections (with video). Gastrointest Endosc 2010;72:1217–25.
12. Bosman FT, Carneiro F, Hruban RH, et al, editors. WHO classification of tumours of the digestive system. Lyon (France): IARC press; 2010.
13. Yamaguchi N, Isomoto H, Fukuda E, et al. Clinical outcomes of endoscopic submucosal dissection for early cancer by indication criteria. Digestion 2009;80:173–81.
14. Gotoda T. Endoscopic resection of early gastric cancer: the Japanese perspective. Curr Opin Gastroenterol 2006;22:561–9.
15. Moehler T, Al-Batran SE, Andus T, et al. German S3-guideline "diagnosis and treatment of esophagogastric cancer". Z Gastroenterol 2011;49:461–531.
16. Hölscher A, Drebber U, Mönig G, et al. Early gastric cancer—lymph node metastasis starts with deep mucosal infiltration. Ann Surg 2009;250:791–7.
17. Isomoto H, Shikuwa S, Yamaguchi N, et al. Endoscopic submucosal dissection for early gastric cancer: a large-scale feasibility study. Gut 2009;58:331–6.
18. Hitomi G, Watanabe H, Tominaga K, et al. Endoscopic submucosal dissection in 100 lesions with early gastric carcinoma. Hepatogastroenterology 2009;56:254–60.
19. Gotoda T, Iwasaki M, Kusano C, et al. Endoscopic resection of early gastric cancer treated by guideline and expanded National Cancer Centre criteria. Br J Surg 2010;97:868–71.
20. Rösch T, Sarbia M, Schumacher B, et al. Attempted endoscopic en bloc resection of mucosal and submucosal tumors using insulated-tip knives: a pilot series. Endoscopy 2004;36:788–801.
21. Neuhaus H, Costamagna G, Devière J, et al. Endoscopic submucosal dissection (ESD) of early neoplastic gastric lesions using a new double-channel endoscope (the "R-scope"). Endoscopy 2006;38:1016–23.
22. Dinis-Ribeiro M, Pimentel-Nunes P, Afonso M, et al. A European case series of endoscopic submucosal dissection for gastric superficial lesions. Gastrointest Endosc 2009;69:350–5.
23. Coda S, Trentino P, Antonellis F, et al. A Western single-center experience with endoscopic submucosal dissection for early gastrointestinal cancers. Gastric Cancer 2010;13:258–63.
24. Probst A, Golger D, Arnholdt H, et al. Endoscopic submucosal dissection of early cancers, flat adenomas, and submucosal tumors in the gastrointestinal tract. Clin Gastroenterol Hepatol 2009;7:149–55.
25. Probst A, Pommer B, Golger D, et al. Endoscopic submucosal dissection in gastric neoplasia—experience from a European center. Endoscopy 2010;42:1037–44.
26. Schumacher B, Charton JP, Nordmann T, et al. Endoscopic submucosal dissection of early gastric neoplasia with a water jet-assisted knife: a Western, single-center experience. Gastrointest Endosc 2012;75:1166–74.

27. Kaehler GF, Sold MG, Fischer K. Selective fluid cushion in the submucosal layer by water jet: advantage for endoscopic mucosal resection. Eur Surg Res 2007; 39:93–7.

28. Schumacher B, Neuhaus H, Enderle MD. Experimental use of new device for mucosectomy. Acta Endoscopica 2007;5:673–8.

29. Neuhaus H, Wirths K, Enderle MD, et al. Randomized controlled study of EMR versus endoscopic submucosal dissection with a water-jet HybridKnife of esophageal lesions in a porcine model. Gastrointest Endosc 2009;70:112–20.

30. Neuhaus H, Schumacher B, Nordmann T, et al. A randomized trial of conventional endoscopic submucosal dissection (CESD) versus water-jet assisted ESD (WESD) of early gastric cancer. Endoscopy 2012;44(Suppl 1):A7.

31. Farhat S, Chaussade S, Ponchon T, et al. Endoscopic submucosal dissection in a European setting. A multi-institutional report of a technique in development. Endoscopy 2011;43:664–70.

32. Ribeiro-Mourao F, Piemental-Nunes P, Dinis-Ribeiro M. Endoscopic submucosal dissection for gastric lesions: results of a European inquiry. Endoscopy 2010;42:814–9.

33. Tajima Y, Nakanishi Y, Ochiai A, et al. Histopathologic findings predicting lymph node metastasis and prognostic of patients with superficial esophageal carcinoma: analysis of 240 surgically resected tumors. Cancer 2000;88:1285–93.

34. Fujishiro M, Yahagi N, Kakushima N, et al. Endoscopic submucosal dissection of esophageal squamous cell neoplasms. Clin Gastroenterol Hepatol 2006;4:688–94.

35. Oyama T, Tomori A, Hotta K, et al. Endoscopic submucosal dissection of early esophageal cancer. Clin Gastroenterol Hepatol 2005;3:67–70.

36. Ishihara R, Iishi H, Uedo N, et al. Comparison of EMR and endoscopic submucosal dissection for en bloc resection of early esophageal cancers in Japan. Gastrointest Endosc 2008;68:1066–72.

37. Deprez PH, Bergman JJ, Meisner S, et al. Current practice with submucosal endoscopic dissection in Europe: position from a panel of experts. Endoscopy 2010;42:853–8.

38. Repici A, Hassan C, Carlino A, et al. Endoscopic submucosal dissection in patients with early esophageal squamous cell carcinoma: results from a prospective Western series. Gastrointest Endosc 2010;71:715–21.

39. Peters FP, Kara MA, Rosmolen WD, et al. Endoscopic treatment of high-grade dysplasia and early stage cancer in Barrett's esophagus. Gastrointest Endosc 2005;61:506–14.

40. Pech O, Behrens A, May A, et al. Long-term results and risk analysis for recurrence after curative endoscopic therapy in 349 patients with high-grade intraepithelial neoplasia and mucosal adenocarcinoma in Barrett's esophagus. Gut 2008;57:1200–6.

41. Pouw RE, Wirths K, Eisendraht P, et al. Efficacy of radiofrequency ablation combined with endoscopic resection for Barrett's esophagus with early neoplasia. Clin Gastroenterol Hepatol 2010;8:23–9.

42. Deprez PH, Piessevaux H, Aouattah T, et al. ESD in Barrett's esophagus high grade dysplasia and mucosal cancer: prospective comparison with CAP mucosectomy. Gastrointest Endosc 2010;71:AB126.

43. Van Vilsteren FG, Pouw RE, Seewald S, et al. Stepwise radical endoscopic resection versus radiofrequency ablation for Barrett's oesophagus with high-grade dysplasia or early cancer: a multicentre randomized trial. Gut 2011;60:765–73.

44. Neuhaus H, Terheggen G, Rutz EM, et al. Endoscopic submucosal dissection plus radiofrequency ablation of neoplastic Barrett's esophagus. Endoscopy 2012;44:1105–13.
45. Buchner AM, Guarner-Argente C, Ginsberg GG. Outcomes of EMR of defiant colorectal lesions directed to an endoscopy referral center. Gastrointest Endosc 2012;76:255–63.
46. Moss A, Bourke MJ, Williams SJ, et al. Endoscopic mucosal resection outcomes and prediction of submucosal cancer from advanced colonic mucosal neoplasia. Gastroenterology 2011;140:1907–18.
47. Pohl J, Borgulya M, Gerges C, et al. Early and late recurrence rates after endoscopic resection of laterally spreading tumors (LST) in the colorectum—a prospective two-center study. Endoscopy 2012;44(Suppl 1):A135.
48. Moss A, Bourke MJ, Williams SJ, et al. Predictors of therapeutic success for endoscopic mucosal resection (EMR) of laterally spreading tumours (LSTs) and large sessile colonic polyps: results of the prospective, multicenter Australian colonic EMR (ACE) study. Gastrointest Endosc 2010;71:AB111.
49. Probst A, Golger D, Anthuber M, et al. Endoscopic submucosal dissection in large sessile lesions of the rectosigmoid: learning curve in a European center. Endoscopy 2012;44:660–7.
50. Repici A, Hassan C, Pagano N, et al. High efficacy of endoscopic submucosal dissection for rectal laterally spreading tumors larger than 3 cm. Gastrointest Endosc 2013;77:96–101.
51. Hochberger J, Maiss J. Currently available simulators: ex vivo models. Gastrointest Endosc Clin N Am 2006;16:435–49.
52. Berr F, Ponchon T, Neureiter D, et al. Experimental endoscopic submucosal dissection training in a porcine model: learning experience of skilled Western endoscopists. Dig Endosc 2011;23:281–9.

ESD Around the World: United States

Norio Fukami, MD

KEYWORDS

- Endoscopic submucosal dissection • Endoscopic training • Learning curve

KEY POINTS

- Main hurdles for adoption of endoscopic submucosal dissection (ESD) in the United States have been the lack of necessary equipment, target lesions suitable for ESD, and training programs.
- ESD demands high technical proficiency and therefore requires a dedicated training program prior to performing ESD in clinical cases.
- Further advancement of techniques and equipment may further facilitate the adoption of ESD by US physicians.

Endoscopic submucosal dissection (ESD) was first reported in Japan in the late 1990s. It quickly gained popularity due to improvement of techniques and available equipment, and before long it spread to other Asian countries. The main indication for ESD in the gastrointestinal tract was early gastric cancer, for which excellent outcomes were reported with endoscopic mucosal resection (EMR) if invasion depth and size were limited.[1]

Many well-trained physicians from the United States have visited high-volume ESD centers in Japan to observe and learn the technique, clearly demonstrating the enthusiasm of American physicians willing to adopt this technique. However, there was originally limited availability of the knives that were developed specifically for the procedure (US Food and Drug Administration [FDA] approval was only achieved later in 2009). Moreover, in North America, there is a lack of target pathology in the gastrointestinal tract (ie, early gastric cancer). In some Asian countries, national mass screening programs have been developed (which started in Japan in 1983 and subsequently in Korea in 1999).[2,3] Gastric cancer screening programs shifted the discovery of gastric cancers to those in early stage, and further endoscopic treatment and surveillance were performed for those patients.[4] In the United States, gastric cancer incidence is lower, and universal screening is not recommended.

Division of Gastroenterology and Hepatology, University of Colorado Anschutz Medical Campus, 12631 East 17th Avenue, B158, Aurora, CO 80045, USA
E-mail address: norio.fukami@ucdenver.edu

Gastrointest Endoscopy Clin N Am 24 (2014) 313–320
http://dx.doi.org/10.1016/j.giec.2013.12.004   giendo.theclinics.com
1052-5157/14/$ – see front matter © 2014 Elsevier Inc. All rights reserved.

Colon cancer is the second leading cause of cancer death in the United States, and mass screening colonoscopy has been shown to improve colon cancer mortality. Large colorectal lesions or intramucosal cancers are usually treated by EMR with proven benefit and efficacy,[5] and in 2001, the Center for Medicare and Medicaid Services approved colonoscopy as the primary screening modality for colorectal cancer. Also, the recent rise in incidence of adenocarcinoma of the esophagus alarmed physicians, and Barrett's related dysplasia surveillance was initiated and is now widely practiced. Nodular dysplasia containing high-grade dysplasia or intramucosal cancer is not an uncommon finding during screening and surveillance endoscopies for Barrett esophagus, and EMR has become the standard diagnostic and therapeutic modality.[6] Naturally, those lesions in the colon and the esophagus would be ideal targets for advanced endoscopic resection (ie, ESD), especially for larger lesions. However, both the colon and esophagus are considered high-risk locations for complications (especially perforation), and therefore in Asia it is recommended to start learning ESD in the stomach.[7,8]

The American Society of Gastrointestinal Endoscopy (ASGE) published a technology status evaluation report on EMR and ESD in 2008,[9] but at the time, coverage of ESD was limited because of unavailability of FDA-approved ESD knives in the United States. Furthermore, there were no training centers in the United States for ESD-specific education, and to date, there are no guidelines on how to be trained in ESD in the United States. Therefore, pilgrimage to Japan (and more recently to Korea or China) continues to be the major pathway for American physicians to learn ESD.

ISSUES FOR ESD TRAINING IN THE UNITED STATES

The lack of training pathways is well recognized as a hurdle for adopting ESD in the United States. Traditional training in Japan consists of learning the basic technical knowledge of ESD (indication, equipment, and techniques), observing expert endoscopists performing ESD in live cases or live demonstration courses, participating in ESD procedures as an assistant (typically 5, but up to 40 cases, providing opportunity for additional learning prior to actually performing ESD), and then finally performing supervised ESD procedure with hands-on assistance from experts. All of these training tiers suggest initiation with gastric neoplasms in the distal third of the stomach, because ESD is technically easier with fewer complications at this location compared with the colon or the esophagus.[10,11]

Several Japanese groups have reported on the gastric ESD learning curve, but opinions vary on the matter, with reports of ESD sufficiency to proficiency requiring experience with 30 to 80 ESDs.[10–16] Thirty cases have been shown to be required for beginners to successfully acquire the ESD techniques,[10,13–15] with en bloc resection rates increasing to 85% from 45% after performance of 40 cases.[12] Excellent clinical outcomes during vigorous, progressive upper ESD training periods have been reported (30 cases, standard resection criteria)[17]; however, further study has shown that trainees must complete 40 to 80 cases to show proficiency at removing difficult lesions, and over 80 cases in order to reach expert level with fewer complications.[11]

The main difficulties for trainees are related to submucosal dissection and control of bleeding.[16] Some training programs aim to minimize these difficulties by incorporating hands-on training using animal models. Before practicing any ESD techniques on humans, either explant tissues or live animal models can be used for practice (**Figs. 1** and **2**).[18,19] The opportunity to practice submucosal dissection is beneficial, but live animal models are needed to simulate the actual human condition of constant luminal wall motions and to practice effective hemostasis during ESD.

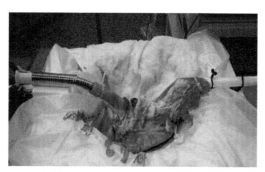

Fig. 1. Explant porcine model for upper ESD practice. (*Courtesy of* Naohisa Yahagi, MD, PhD, Tokyo, Japan.)

Currently, only a handful of physicians perform ESD routinely in the United States, while expert endoscopists are more readily available in Japan. Because practice opportunities under direct supervision are not as abundant here, animal model training would be the preferred method to train physicians in the United States. In fact, in low-volume centers in both Europe and South America, use of a porcine model for practicing ESD without expert supervision has been shown to strengthen technical skills.[18–22] Regardless of whether it is to include animal model training or not, the step-wise method of learning ESD that has been established in Japan should be adopted by physicians in the United States.

Another setback to widespread use of ESD in the United States is the infrequent finding of early gastric cancer. The standard Japanese model for learning ESD, which

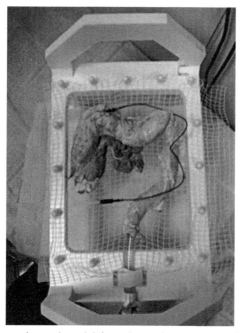

Fig. 2. Explant bovine colorectal model for colorectal ESD practice. (*Courtesy of* Naohisa Yahagi, MD, PhD, Tokyo, Japan.)

is to gain proficiency in gastric ESD before attempting either the colon or the esophagus, is not feasible here. Although not yet established, a direct approach to organ-specific ESD training would be more beneficial in the United States. For instance, Iacopini and colleagues[23] have shown a potential method for fast-track training of colonic ESD. An experienced endoscopist (ESD trainee) first performed five ESDs on explant porcine stomach, without the supervision of an expert, before traveling to an expert center to observe 40 gastric and colonic ESDs. After the observation period, the trainee performed one ESD similar to his original practice, but this time under the supervision of his expert trainer. This same trainer then supervised the performance of one rectal ESD procedure (retraining at 11th procedure). The en bloc resection rate reached 80% after five procedures in the rectum and after 20 procedures in the colon. This study suggested that colorectal ESD can be successfully learned after training in an explant stomach model. It should be noted that colonic ESD was only performed after achieving 80% en bloc resection rate in the rectum.

Adequate preclinical training is extremely important, as complications during ESD can be severe, possibly resulting in need for surgery, and an inability to achieve en bloc resection would nullify the clinical benefit of ESD. ESD is technically demanding, and even experienced endoscopists face high complication rates as they begin learning ESD. In fact, when a large group of ESD-novice Asian endoscopists was trained in ESD using a porcine model during an effort to examine the main difficulties experienced during training, bleeding and perforation occurred in over half of the cases (56% and 65%, respectively),[24] proving that learning ESD is difficult, and not only for those in the West.

CURRENT MOVES AND THE FUTURE OF ESD TRAINING IN THE UNITED STATES

Many institutions are moving forward with self-structured ESD training programs using explant and live animal models. To make this happen, physicians are either hosting a guest trainer (eg, Japanese expert) or have themselves visited expert ESD centers outside the country and observed many cases to learn the technique, then self-started ESD practice to gain more experience. It is exciting that some physicians are taking this initiative, the first step to acquiring the technique of ESD; however, there are currently no guidelines in the United States regarding when to start clinical practice of ESD on humans, and this lack of a uniform approach poses a potentially significant problem in regards to the quality of patient care and outcome. The author has mentored several physicians in the United States in their hands-on training with animal models and by proctoring when they start ESD in human cases, with appropriate privileges to perform such endoscopic procedures at those specific institutions. They have been successful in starting clinical practice of ESD (personal communication), and therefore this could be another model in the United States for spreading the use of ESD to benefit patients with acceptable risks and outcomes. The necessity for high quality preclinical practice using animal models cannot be stressed enough to achieve proficiency at ESD, and there is an urgent need for training courses in the United States.

To overcome the lack of training opportunities for various endoscopic techniques, the ASGE has been hosting educational or refresher-type hands-on courses, including dedicated multiday courses with an emphasis on providing both cognitive and hands-on components and exposure-type hands-on only courses at the national meetings **Figs. 3** and **4**. Recently, the ASGE has begun planning a new training certificate program called Skills Training Assessment Reinforcement (STAR) (http://www.asge.org/education/education.aspx?id=16755). The initial course's focus is on EMR, and a

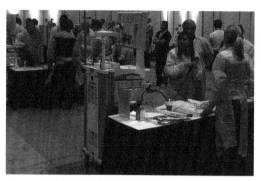

Fig. 3. EMR/ESD hands-on training session at Digestive Disease Week 2013.

certificate of attendance is awarded once the trainee passes the assessment. Training is performed at the ASGE's newly built, state-of-the-art Institute for Training & Technology (IT&T Center), where both lectures and technical components using explant and live animals can be taught. It is hoped that this program will expand to ESD training in the future.

The ASGE successfully hosted the first North American ESD course at the aforementioned IT&T center in December 2013. This course received outstanding feedback for both the structure of the course and the quality of trainers. The hands-on training portion began with explant porcine models and then live pig models for further practice of ESD in an environment similar to actual human cases. Furthermore, in 2012 the ASGE initiated a special interest group (SIG) for ASGE members enthusiastic about ESD, and with adequate support from the members the ESD SIG was officially approved in 2013.

Yet another barrier to the widespread use of ESD in the United States is the lack of an appropriate billing code for this highly intensive and time-consuming procedure. However, as seen in Japan, this procedure would benefit those patients who may be cured by minimally invasive endoscopic procedures rather than surgical resection, which would reduce not only overall cost but also morbidity and mortality. The movement to obtain an appropriate code for ESD would require collaborative effort on the part of patients, physicians, and the societies of gastrointestinal disease and

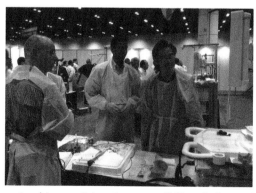

Fig. 4. Dr Haru Inoue teaching participants on cap EMR technique using explant porcine model.

endoscopy, but would be worth it in order to ensure this highly effective and beneficial procedure becomes more widely practiced.

ADVANCEMENT OF ESD TO FURTHER LOWER THE HURDLE

Additional modifications of technique and equipment may assist the spread of ESD. As discussed previously, the high degree of technical difficulty to acquire proficiency has been a major issue. To reduce this difficulty, several new techniques have been proposed (circumferential marginal incision and snare resection; simplified or hybrid ESD[25,26] and balloon-assisted submucosal dissection; submucosal endoscopy with mucosal resection[27,28]; and countertraction using various methods[29]). New submucosal fluid cushion materials have been investigated in animal models in the United States; there are several that assist ESD by creating a long-lasting cushion,[30,31] and another type that promotes chemical dissociation of disulfide bonds, thereby reducing the resistance of the submucosa during dissection.[32] Hopefully the advancement of techniques and materials will assist the dissemination of ESD in the United States.

SUMMARY

ESD is well accepted as an advanced mucosal resection technique in most Asian countries; however, it demands highly advanced technical skills in addition to thorough training in pretreatment diagnosis, knowledge of equipment features, and the capability to effectively treat possible complications. ESD could be a promising treatment modality for the United States, and yet it is vastly underutilized because of many obstacles. Possible solutions are slowly arising, however, and a concerted effort to more widely disseminate ESD from both physicians and the societies of gastroenterology and gastrointestinal endoscopy could potentially benefit many of those patients for whom ESD could offer a cure without invasive surgery.

ACKNOWLEDGMENTS

The author would like to express deep appreciation to Alissa Bults, MS, for her dedication and significant contribution to this article and this issue of ESD.

REFERENCES

1. Shen L, Shan YS, Hu HM, et al. Management of gastric cancer in Asia: resource-stratified guidelines. Lancet Oncol 2013;14:535–47.
2. Hamashima C, Shibuya D, Yamazaki H, et al. The Japanese guidelines for gastric cancer screening. Jpn J Clin Oncol 2008;38:259–67.
3. Lee KS, Oh DK, Han MA, et al. Gastric cancer screening in Korea: report on the national cancer screening program in 2008. Cancer Res Treat 2011;43: 83–8.
4. Chung SJ, Park MJ, Kang SJ, et al. Effect of annual endoscopic screening on clinicopathologic characteristics and treatment modality of gastric cancer in a high-incidence region of Korea. Int J Cancer 2012;131:2376–84.
5. Levin B, Lieberman DA, McFarland B, et al. Screening and surveillance for the early detection of colorectal cancer and adenomatous polyps, 2008: a joint guideline from the American Cancer Society, the US Multi-Society Task Force on Colorectal Cancer, and the American College of Radiology. Gastroenterology 2008;134:1570–95.

6. Spechler SJ, Sharma P, Souza RF, et al. American Gastroenterological Association technical review on the management of Barrett's esophagus. Gastroenterology 2011;140:18–52.

7. Goda K, Fujishiro M, Hirasawa T, et al. How to teach and learn endoscopic submucosal dissection for upper gastrointestinal neoplasm in Japan. Dig Endosc 2012;24:136–42.

8. Tanaka S, Tamegai Y, Tsuda S, et al. Multicenter questionnaire survey on the current situation of colorectal endoscopic submucosal dissection in Japan. Dig Endosc 2010;22:S2–8.

9. ASGE Technology Committee, Kantsevoy SV, Adler DG, Conway JD, et al. Endoscopic mucosal resection and endoscopic submucosal dissection. Gastrointest Endosc 2008;68:11–8.

10. Gotoda T, Friedland S, Hamanaka H, et al. A learning curve for advanced endoscopic resection. Gastrointest Endosc 2005;62:866–7.

11. Yamamoto Y, Fujisaki J, Ishiyama A, et al. Current status of training for endoscopic submucosal dissection for gastric epithelial neoplasm at Cancer Institute Hospital, Japanese Foundation for Cancer Research, a famous Japanese hospital. Dig Endosc 2012;24:6.

12. Choi IJ, Kim CG, Chang HJ, et al. The learning curve for EMR with circumferential mucosal incision in treating intramucosal gastric neoplasm. Gastrointest Endosc 2005;62:860–5.

13. Kakushima N, Fujishiro M, Kodashima S, et al. A learning curve for endoscopic submucosal dissection of gastric epithelial neoplasms. Endoscopy 2006;38:991–5.

14. Kato M, Gromski M, Jung Y, et al. The learning curve for endoscopic submucosal dissection in an established experimental setting. Surg Endosc 2013;27:154–61.

15. Oda I, Odagaki T, Suzuki H, et al. Learning curve for endoscopic submucosal dissection of early gastric cancer based on trainee experience. Dig Endosc 2012;24:129–32.

16. Yamamoto S, Uedo N, Ishihara R, et al. Endoscopic submucosal dissection for early gastric cancer performed by supervised residents: assessment of feasibility and learning curve. Endoscopy 2009;41:923–8.

17. Tsuji Y, Ohata K, Sekiguchi M, et al. An effective training system for endoscopic submucosal dissection of gastric neoplasm. Endoscopy 2011;43:1033–8.

18. Parra-Blanco A, Arnau MR, Nicolas-Perez D, et al. Endoscopic submucosal dissection training with pig models in a Western country. World J Gastroenterol 2010;16:2895–900.

19. Berr F, Ponchon T, Neureiter D, et al. Experimental endoscopic submucosal dissection training in a porcine model: learning experience of skilled Western endoscopists. Dig Endosc 2011;23:281–9.

20. Vazquez-Sequeiros E, de Miquel DB, Olcina JR, et al. Training model for teaching endoscopic submucosal dissection of gastric tumors. Rev Esp Enferm Dig 2009;101:546–52.

21. Parra-Blanco A, Gonzalez C, Arnau MR. Ex vivo and in vivo models for endoscopic submucosal dissection training. Clin Endosc 2012;45:350–7.

22. Othman MO, Wallace MB. Endoscopic mucosal resection (EMR) and endoscopic submucosal dissection (ESD) in 2011, a Western perspective. Clin Res Hepatol Gastroenterol 2011;35:288–94.

23. Iacopini F, Bella A, Costamagna G, et al. Stepwise training in rectal and colonic endoscopic submucosal dissection with differentiated learning curves. Gastrointest Endosc 2012;76:1188–96.

24. Teoh A, Chiu P, Wong S, et al. Difficulties and outcomes in starting endoscopic submucosal dissection. Surg Endosc 2010;24:1049–54.

25. Toyonaga T, Man IM, Morita Y, et al. The new resources of treatment for early stage colorectal tumors: EMR with small incision and simplified endoscopic submucosal dissection. Dig Endosc 2009;21:S31–7.

26. Moss A, Bourke MJ, Metz AJ, et al. Beyond the snare: technically accessible large en bloc colonic resection in the West: an animal study. Dig Endosc 2012; 24:21–9.

27. Takizawa K, Knipschield MA, Gostout CJ. Submucosal endoscopy with mucosal resection (SEMR): a new hybrid technique of endoscopic submucosal balloon dissection in the porcine rectosigmoid colon. Surg Endosc 2013;27:4457–62.

28. Gostout CJ, Knipschield MA. Submucosal endoscopy with mucosal resection: a hybrid endoscopic submucosal dissection in the porcine rectum and distal colon. Gastrointest Endosc 2012;76:829–34.

29. Fukami N. What we want for ESD is a second hand! Traction method. Gastrointest Endosc 2013;78:274–6.

30. Feitoza AB, Gostout CJ, Burgart LJ, et al. Hydroxypropyl methylcellulose: a better submucosal fluid cushion for endoscopic mucosal resection. Gastrointest Endosc 2003;57:41–7.

31. Khashab MA, Saxena P, Sharaiha RZ, et al. A novel submucosal gel permits simple and efficient gastric endoscopic submucosal dissection. Gastroenterology 2013;144:505–7.

32. Sumiyama K, Gostout CJ, Rajan E, et al. Chemically assisted endoscopic mechanical submucosal dissection by using mesna. Gastrointest Endosc 2008;67: 534–8.

Index

Note: Page numbers of article titles are in **boldface** type.

Gastrointest Endoscopy Clin N Am 24 (2014) 321–325
http://dx.doi.org/10.1016/S1052-5157(14)00011-7
1052-5157/14/$ – see front matter © 2014 Elsevier Inc. All rights reserved.

giendo.theclinics.com

Moving?

Make sure your subscription moves with you!

To notify us of your new address, find your **Clinics Account Number** (located on your mailing label above your name), and contact customer service at:

Email: journalscustomerservice-usa@elsevier.com

800-654-2452 (subscribers in the U.S. & Canada)
314-447-8871 (subscribers outside of the U.S. & Canada)

Fax number: 314-447-8029

Elsevier Health Sciences Division
Subscription Customer Service
3251 Riverport Lane
Maryland Heights, MO 63043

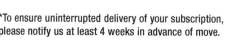
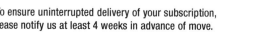

Printed and bound by CPI Group (UK) Ltd, Croydon, CR0 4YY

03/10/2024

01040496-0017